ωωιμι ci) 43431

-2 NOV. 2004

2·12·04·

28. JUL. 2005

-5. SEP. 2005

-4. NOV. 2005

15, 12-05

-9. MAY 2006

26 MAY 2006

15 SEP 2006

24. NOV. 2006

31. JAN. 2007

28. AUG. 2007

4. OCT. 2007

24. OCT. 2007

8. SEP. 2008

26. AUG. 2010

23 JAN 2013

This book should be returned by the last date
stamped above. You may renew the loan
personally, by post or telephone for a further
period if the book is not required by
another reader.

D1426992

IIII 2004

Manual of Eye Emergencies

Diagnosis and Management

To Clemency, Douglas, Duncan and James

For Butterworth-Heinemann

Publishing Director: Caroline Makepeace
Development Editor: Kim Benson
Project Manager: Joannah Duncan
Designer: George Ajayi

Manual of Eye Emergencies

Diagnosis and Management

Lennox A. Webb MBChB FRCS FRCOphth
Consultant Ophthalmic Surgeon, Royal Alexandra Hospital,
Paisley, UK

Foreword by

Jack J. Kanski MD MS FRCS FRCOphth
Honorary Consultant Ophthalmic Surgeon, Prince Charles Eye Unit,
King Edward VII Hospital, Windsor, UK

BUTTERWORTH
HEINEMANN

Edinburgh London New York Oxford Philadelphia St Louis Sydney Toronto 2004

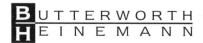

BUTTERWORTH-HEINEMANN
An imprint of Elsevier Limited

First edition 1995
Second edition 2004

ISBN 0 7506 5219 5

British Library Cataloguing in Publication Data
A catalogue record for this book is available from the British Library

Library of Congress Cataloging in Publication Data
A catalog record for this book is available from the Library of Congress

Note
Medical knowledge is constantly changing. Standard safety precautions must be
followed, but as new research and clinical experience broaden our knowledge,
changes in treatment and drug therapy may become necessary or appropriate.
Readers are advised to check the most current product information provided by
the manufacturer of each drug to be administered to verify the recommended
dose, the method and duration of administration, and contraindications. It is the
responsibility of the practitioner, relying on experience and knowledge of the
patient, to determine dosages and the best treatment for each individual patient.
Neither the Publisher nor the author assumes any liability for any injury and/or
damage to persons or property arising from this publication.

Printed in China

Contents

Foreword

This practical and pragmatic book has been written for those who may have little knowledge of ophthalmology, but who are required to diagnose and manage eye patients.

The text concentrates largely on common eye problems, and is designed to lead the clinician towards the likely diagnosis and most appropriate management. The majority of surgical procedures used in ophthalmology are described briefly and some simple techniques are illustrated in detail as a guide for suitably qualified clinician.

With its emphasis on guiding the user towards safe and effective management of common eye conditions, this book is an extremely valuable tool for any professional involved in primary eye care.

Jack Kanski, 2004

Preface

This book assumes the reader has little knowledge of ophthalmology, and acts as a guide to the most appropriate diagnosis and management of the majority of common eye complaints. Intentionally it does not enter into detailed discussion, but concentrates on the practical initial treatment and referral pathway. Extensive cross-referencing is used to allow fast navigation, and practical charts and pictures can be used directly from this book, to test patients' visual function, or to help identify their medication. Repetition, where this occurs, is deliberate to allow rapid access to management pathways. Most eye problems are not true emergencies, but are perceived to be so by both patients and practitioners, hence the title of this book.

Lennox A. Webb, 2004

Chapter 1

Basic Examination

History

An accurate and detailed history often points to the diagnosis and guides your examination.

BASIC EXAMINATION (Fig. 1.1)

The basic examination should cover the following.

Face, Lids and Orbit

External Appearance (Fig. 1.2)

- eczema, trauma, cellulitis, allergic responses, styes, cysts, tumors, proptosis.

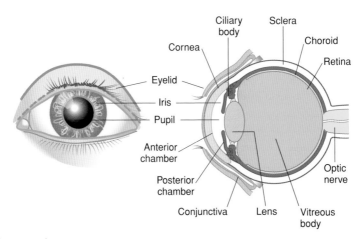

Fig. 1.1 The eye.

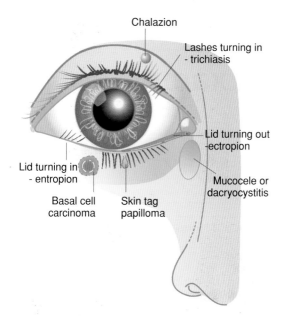

Fig. 1.2 The eye – external appearance.

If patient is unable to open eyes due to pain – instill a drop of local anesthetic into each eye – proxymetacaine 0.5% or similar – this may allow you to continue examination if pain is from surface trauma.

Visual Acuity (VA) (Figs 1.3, 1.4)

- always document this for each eye **individually** – the patient may have perfect vision in one eye and be blind in the other
- range of distance visual acuity:

NPL	No Perception of Light
HM	Hand Movements only
CF	able to Count Fingers held in front of face
6/60–6/4	as read from Snellen chart

- use correct glasses (distance and **not** reading glasses for a 6 meter Snellen visual acuity) or contact lenses if usually worn
- use a pinhole if vision is reduced (Fig. 1.5).

What is a Pinhole?

As stated, simply a small hole or group of holes in a piece of card or plastic, which corrects visual acuity to approximately that achieved with glasses (Figs 1.5 and 1.6); make one by pushing a needle through the back cover of this book.

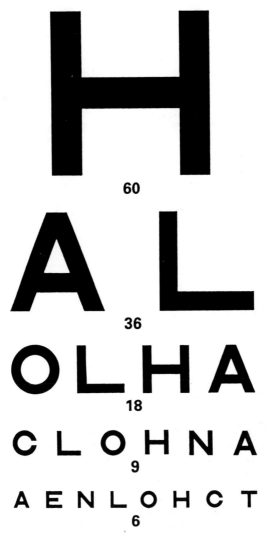

Fig. 1.3 Visual acuity chart. Use the above chart from 3 meters with **distance** glasses if worn.

Normal Vision is 6/6 (or 20/20)

If vision is reduced, document carefully and refer to Chapter 4, page 73.

TEST TYPES

N.5.

Now we have reached the trees—the beautiful trees! never so beautiful as to-day. Imagine the effect of a straight and regular double avenue of oaks, nearly a mile long, arching over-head, and closing into perspective like the roof and columns of a cathedral. every tree and branch encrusted with the bright and delicate congelation of hoar-frost, white and pure as snow, delicate and defined as carved ivory. How
— numerous renew assurance our sense ewe camera acorn assess cocoa source essence err —

N.8.

a wide view over four counties—a landscape of snow. A deep lane leads abruptly down the hill; a mere narrow cart-track, sinking between high banks clothed with fern and furze and low broom, crowned with luxuriant
— cam macaroon overseas race ocean excess nurse answer raven —

N.12.

this is rime in its loveliest form ! And there is still a berry here and there on the holly, "blushing in its natural coral," through the delicate tracery,
— same accrue car oxen recover ensnare —

N.18.

wren, "that shadow of a bird," as White, of Selbourne, calls it,
— severe room caravan —

N.36.

amongst the
— occur —

Fig. 1.4   Reading visual acuity chart. Use **reading** glasses if worn.

How is Vision Documented?

■ the top number is the distance in meters from the test chart, the bottom number is the distance at which a normally sighted person would be able to read the test. So if the patient can only read down to the 6/18 line (ensure they are at the appropriate distance, and wearing distance glasses if required) document '6/18' RE (right eye) or LE (left eye) as appropriate. This indicates that this patient can only see at 6 meters what a normally sighted person could see at 18 meters, so the patient's vision is subnormal (Fig. 1.7).

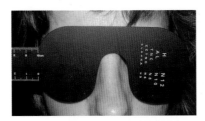

Fig. 1.5 Using a pinhole.

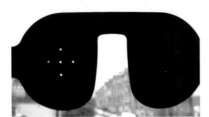

Fig. 1.6 Pinhole.

VA 6/18

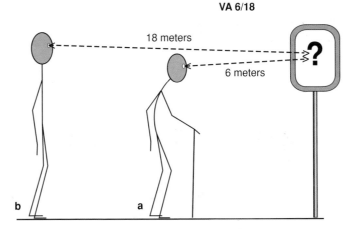

Fig. 1.7 Patient with reduced vision (a) has to stand at 6 meters to see same object that normal-sighted individual (b) can see at 18 meters = 6/18 vision.

Eye Movements

- if defective and of sudden onset the patient may complain of double vision (see Fig. 1.10)
- use a pentorch or pencil at least 2 feet from the patient, tell them to keep their head still (hold it if required), and ask them to follow the light as you move it to the six positions shown in Fig. 1.8
- ask if they see double when looking straight ahead

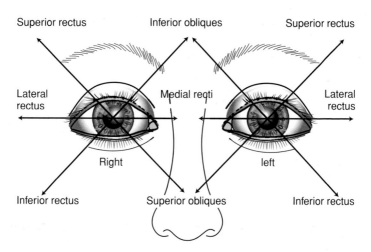

Fig. 1.8   Direction of action of extraocular muscles.

- if yes, are the two images side to side (horizontal diplopia) or one above the other (vertical diplopia) (see p. 107 and Figs 1.9 and 1.10)
- do they see double in any other position of gaze – if so this points to which muscle is weak or restricted.

Conjunctiva and Sclera

Look for injection, hemorrhage and discharge.

Cornea

- this should be clear with a bright smooth surface (Fig. 1.11)

Fig. 1.9   Vertical diplopia.

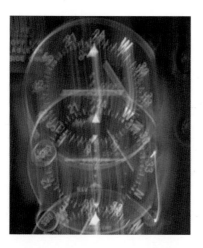

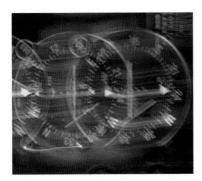

Fig. 1.10 Horizontal diplopia.

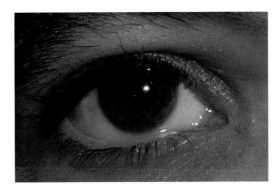

Fig. 1.11 Normal cornea with normal light reflex.

- if you suspect a corneal injury stain with fluorescein drops and look for abrasions (see Fig. 2.3), foreign bodies, which may be subtarsal (underneath the upper lid) (see Fig. 2.12), and evidence of perforation (see Fig. 2.13a).

Pupils

- should be round, equal in size and react briskly to a bright light
- in the elderly the pupil is often smaller and reacts sluggishly
- look for an afferent pupil defect (APD – see below) which may be present even with normal visual acuity
- check the red reflex (see below).

What is an Afferent Pupillary Defect (APD)?

- this occurs when the pupil enlarges rather than contracts when a light is shone into the affected eye
- it is caused by a defect in optic nerve transmission either due to inflammation (as with optic neuritis), optic nerve damage, or gross reduction in retinal function.

How to Check for an APD

- shine a bright light for 2 seconds into one pupil, then switch briskly to the other side again for 2 full seconds
- do not do it faster, or you may miss the sign
- if one pupil dilates as you shine the light at it, an afferent defect is present.

Red Reflex (Fig. 1.12)

This is the reflex seen from the retina when a light is shone through the pupil, as seen in flash photos, when this appears as a 'red eye'; look through an ophthalmoscope at the pupil from about 18 inches – opacities or surface irregularities such as cataract, vitreous hemorrhage and corneal abrasions block or reduce this reflex; a white reflex in an infant may indicate a retinoblastoma (rare).

Fundus (Retina) (Figs 1.13 and 1.14)

You should attempt to observe three regions with a direct ophthalmoscope

1. **Optic disc** for cupping, pallor, swelling and hemorrhages
2. **Central retina** for hemorrhages, pallor, atrophy and pigment clumping
3. **Peripheral retina** for hemorrhages, appearance of vessels and retinal detachment.

It may be very difficult to see any details due to a very small pupil, cataract or vitreous hemorrhage (document the fact if no view is visible).

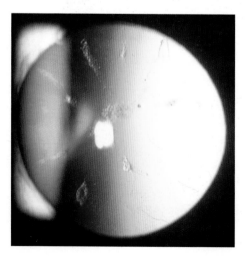

Fig. 1.12 Red reflex – reflected light from retinal surface. The faint opacities are early cataract.

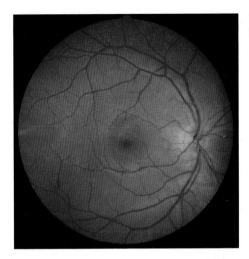

Fig. 1.13 Normal fundus (retina).

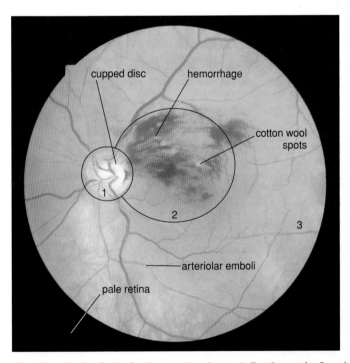

cupped disc   hemorrhage

cotton wool spots

1

2

3

arteriolar emboli

pale retina

Fig. 1.14 Fundus (retina). Observe 3 regions – 1 disc, 2 macula, 3 periphery.

Visual Fields (Fig. 1.15)

A quick screen is all that is required in those with suspected neuropathology.

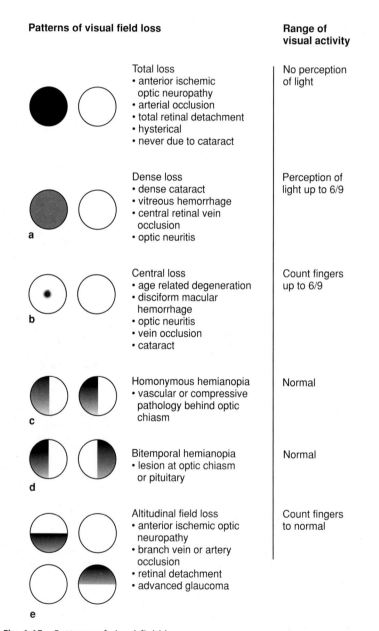

Patterns of visual field loss

Range of visual activity

Total loss
- anterior ischemic optic neuropathy
- arterial occlusion
- total retinal detachment
- hysterical
- never due to cataract

No perception of light

Dense loss
- dense cataract
- vitreous hemorrhage
- central retinal vein occlusion
- optic neuritis

Perception of light up to 6/9

a

Central loss
- age related degeneration
- disciform macular hemorrhage
- optic neuritis
- vein occlusion
- cataract

Count fingers up to 6/9

b

Homonymous hemianopia
- vascular or compressive pathology behind optic chiasm

Normal

c

Bitemporal hemianopia
- lesion at optic chiasm or pituitary

Normal

d

Altitudinal field loss
- anterior ischemic optic neuropathy
- branch vein or artery occlusion
- retinal detachment
- advanced glaucoma

Count fingers to normal

e

Fig. 1.15   Patterns of visual field loss.

1. Sit directly facing the patient at 1 meter.
2. Instruct patient to cover one eye – without pressing it – and look straight into your eye on the same side, the patient's left eye looking into your right and vice-versa.
3. Ensure that the patient keeps fixing on your eye – important as the test is invalid otherwise – and ask if they are aware of your hair, nose, mouth, neck, collar – if yes, central vision is grossly intact.

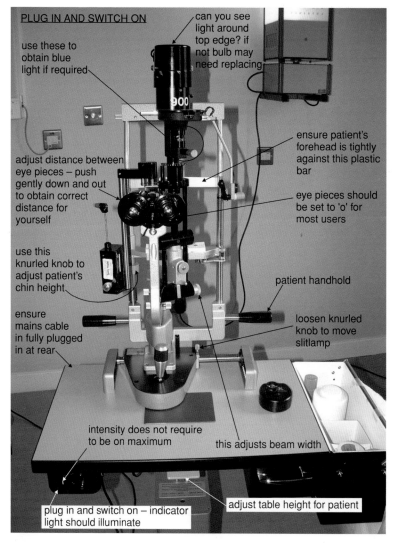

Fig. 1.16 Slit lamp.

4. Hold an outstretched index finger in each field quadrant, move it slightly and ask if the patient sees this movement – move in centrally until they do.
5. To the side, the patient should see an object in the same plane as their own eyes whilst looking straight ahead.

This is only a basic test of visual fields but is sufficient in a casualty setting.

Pitfalls

Medicolegal problems may arise if you fail to:

- carefully document the history, the fact that you have adequately examined the patient, and your clinical findings
- check visual acuity in each eye individually and document this
- look for evidence of penetrating injury if there is any suspicion of this, or if in doubt, refer
- X-ray cases of trauma involving metal, glass, stone, etc.

Tips on Using the Slit Lamp (Fig. 1.16)

1. Make sure it is plugged in and switched on at the wall, and at the machine.
2. The patient should have their chin firmly on the chin rest, and their forehead right up against the forehead rest.
3. Adjust the height of the lamp to suit the patient – the Haag–Streit slit lamp has a height adjuster lever just under the front of the table mount.
4. The brightness control is adjacent to the on–off switch – start on a low setting initially.
5. A silver, knurled knob near the top of the machine controls the height of the slit beam and the blue light for looking at the cornea after staining with fluorescein.

Chapter 2

Red Eye

Chemical Injury

Wash eye immediately (see p. 112).

Which Category Applies?

- sudden onset, painful

unilateral	p. 17
bilateral	p. 45

- sudden onset, painless

unilateral	p. 55
bilateral	p. 59

■ chronic	p. 62
■ trauma	p. 112

An accurate history will frequently give you the diagnosis before examination.

Most Commonly Due to:

Conjunctivitis (Fig. 2.1)
- diffuse injection with purulent discharge.

Corneal Foreign Body (Fig. 2.2)
- eye may look quiet initially – rust ring with iron particles may develop within hours.

Corneal Abrasion – without Fluorescein Staining (Fig. 2.3a,b)
- the irregular corneal light reflex indicates surface damage – and the edge of the abrasion can be seen.

Corneal Abrasion – with Fluorescein Staining (Fig. 2.3c)
- defect stains vividly.

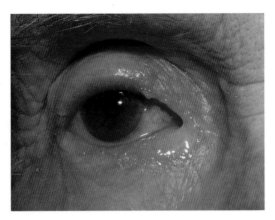

Fig. 2.1   Conjunctivitis.

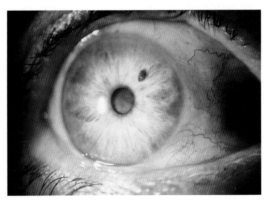

Fig. 2.2   Corneal foreign body.

Ingrowing Eyelashes and Entropion (Fig. 2.4)
■ the lid has turned in allowing lashes to abrade the eye.

Subconjunctival Hemorrhage (Fig. 2.5)
■ dense solid hemorrhage with well-defined edge – may cover whole conjunctiva.

Anterior Uveitis or Iritis (Fig. 2.6)
■ injected especially around the corneal edge (limbus) – eye is very light sensitive (photophobic) and waters – but no purulent discharge.

Allergy
■ main feature is excoriated skin – typical of allergy to eye drops (Fig. 2.7a).

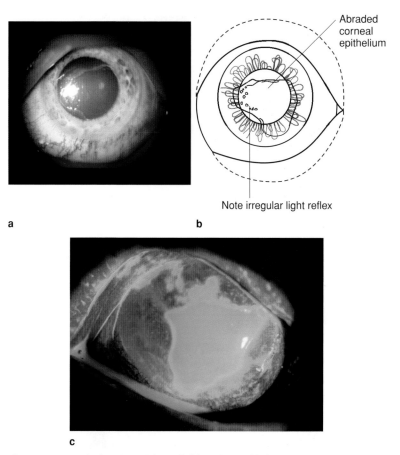

Fig. 2.3 Corneal abrasion without (a,b) and with (c) fluorescein staining.

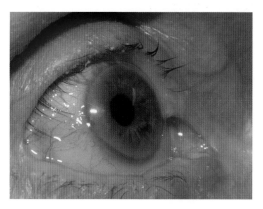

Fig. 2.4 Ingrowing eyelashes and entropion, upper lid.

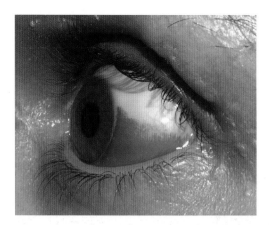

Fig. 2.5   Subconjunctival hemorrhage.

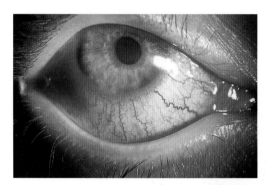

Fig. 2.6   Anterior uveitis/iritis.

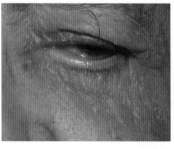

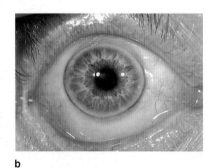

a

b

Fig. 2.7a,b   Allergy.

■ swollen edematous conjunctiva – typical acute response to allergen such as dust (Fig. 2.7b).

Trauma (Fig. 2.8)
■ gross subconjunctival hemorrhage may mask underlying globe rupture.

Corneal Ulcer (Fig. 2.9)
■ this may occur at the corneal margin as shown or more centrally.

Previous Eye Surgery (Fig. 2.10)
■ intraocular infection – endophthalmitis – note pus level in anterior chamber (hypopyon).

Periorbital and Orbital Cellulitis (Fig. 2.11a)
■ underlying eye may also be engorged in orbital cellulitis.

RED EYE – ACUTE ONSET, PAINFUL, UNILATERAL

Common Causes

Corneal abrasion	p. 24
Corneal foreign body (FB)	p. 27

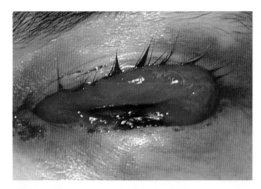

Fig. 2.8 Trauma with gross conjunctival edema and hemorrhage.

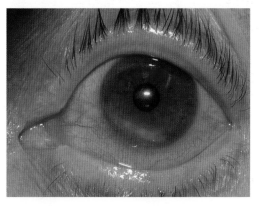

Fig. 2.9 Peripheral corneal ulcer.

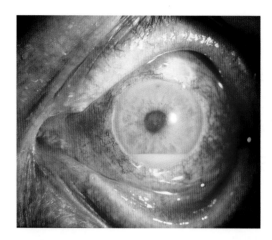

Fig. 2.10 Previous eye surgery – endophthalmitis with hypopyon.

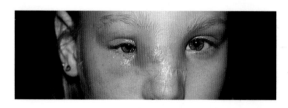

Fig. 2.11a Periorbital and orbital cellulitis.

Less Common Causes

Ask Directly

- **drilling, grinding, welding or hammering.** Look for corneal foreign bodies and consider penetrating injury with high energy particles – usually hammering metal on metal (Fig. 2.11c).
- **painful to look at light (photophobia).** Suggests inflammation within the eye, as with uveitis and severe abrasions.

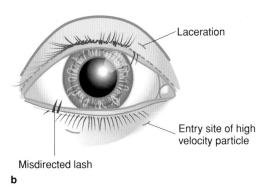

b

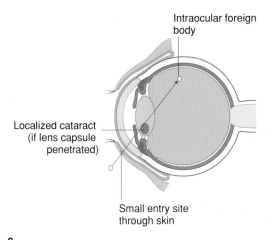

c

Fig. 2.11b,c Lid examination.

- **trauma to the eye – past or present.** Corneal abrasions are frequently caused by an infant's fingernail, newspapers and foreign bodies; previous abrasions may recurrently break down, usually on awakening from sleep. Direct recent trauma is usually easily apparent.
- **contact lenses.** Overwear or poor contact lens hygiene may lead to corneal abrasions or ulcers.
- **eye surgery – recent or past.** Any sudden deterioration after surgery may indicate infection; irritation due to sutures may follow cataract surgery, but is now much less common with the use of modern suture-free surgery; discomfort immediately following retinal detachment and squint surgery is common but soon resolves.
- **previous uveitis ('eye inflammation').** Young men with ankylosing spondylitis often have recurrent uveitis.

■ **reduced vision.** Occurs in most cases, often due to excess watering, photophobia, or disruption of the central optical zone by an abrasion; acute glaucoma causes corneal clouding and occurs predominantly in the elderly.

Examination

Orbit and Periorbital Tissues
1. Document periorbital bruising or erythema.
2. Feel the orbital rim for tenderness or rim fractures (Fig. 2.11d).
3. Document whether protective eyewear was worn if relevant.

Lids
1. Look for misdirected lashes, lacerations or site of entry of high velocity particles (Fig. 2.11b,c).
2. Evert the lid (see p. 32) and look for subtarsal foreign bodies, but **not** if a penetrating injury is suspected.

Visual Acuity (VA)
1. Patient may be unable to open eye due to pain and photophobia – if so …
2. Instill a drop of topical anesthetic, such as proxymetacaine 0.5% – this may allow you to continue the examination.
3. **Do not try to force the lids open** – if a penetrating injury is suspected (see p. 125)
4. Use glasses if appropriate or pinhole (Fig. 1.5).
5. Vision usually reduced with corneal abrasion, contact lens overwear and acute glaucoma – often only minimally reduced with corneal foreign bodies, uveitis or episcleritis.
6. Penetrating injury may lead to either gross or no visual loss depending upon the degree of intraocular damage – see pitfalls on p. 131.

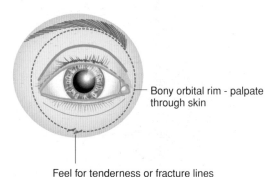

Bony orbital rim - palpate through skin

Feel for tenderness or fracture lines

Fig. 2.11d Examination of periorbital tissues.

Pupil

1. Constriction common in uveitis and corneal abrasions due to pupillary spasm – this is often the source of eye pain, hence the use of relaxants such as cyclopentolate 1%.
2. Fixed oval pupil, hazy cornea, elderly patient, assume acute glaucoma (see p. 41).
3. Distorted pupil, history of trauma, assume penetrating injury.

Conjunctiva

1. Conjunctival hemorrhage or chemosis (edematous swelling) (Figs 2.8, 2.7b) may mask an underlying scleral rupture, localized inflammation suggests episcleritis.
2. Circumferential conjunctival injection near the cornea in the presence of photophobia suggests uveitis (Fig. 2.6).
3. Examine the conjunctival fornices (gutter between inside of eyelids and eye) for foreign bodies, including contact lenses – evert the upper lid (technique, see Figs 2.25–2.28).

Cornea

1. Highlight pathology – usually abrasion, ulcer or foreign body with dilute fluorescein.
2. Foreign bodies may be subtarsal (under the upper eyelid) – giveaway is presence of upper corneal vertical linear scratches (Fig. 2.12) – examine under the upper eyelid (see Figs 2.25–2.28).
3. A distorted pupil indicates a penetrating injury of the cornea or sclera (Fig. 5.11) – to examine for leaking aqueous instill 2% fluorescein and

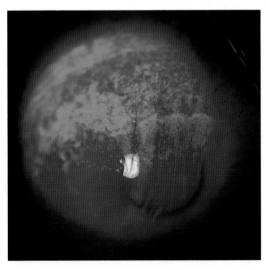

Fig. 2.12 Typical linear corneal abrasions indicating a subtarsal foreign body.

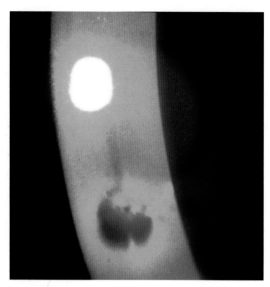

Fig. 2.13a Aqueous leaking from anterior chamber following a perforating injury – seen with fluorescein 2%.

observe under a blue light (Fig. 2.13a); however absence of a leak does not rule out penetrating injury, as the wound may self seal.
4. Hazy cornea, elderly patient, general debility, extreme eye pain and visual loss suggests acute glaucoma (see p. 41).
5. White spots on the inside corneal surface may be seen in uveitis (keratic precipitates) (Fig. 2.14).

Sclera
1. Scleral injection in an acutely tender eye (Fig. 2.15a) suggests uveitis or scleritis. Scleritis is rare – the pain characteristically keeps the patient awake at night.
2. Episcleritis is associated with mild discomfort only.

Anterior Chamber
The anterior chamber is the space between the pupil and the inside surface of the cornea (Fig. 2.13b).

1. Uveitis – haze, which may be very subtle, with inflammatory cells may be visible in the aqueous with a slit lamp.
2. Hyphema – blood level – in trauma may be minimal or fill the whole chamber (Figs 2.15b, 5.4).
3. Hypopyon – white level of inflammatory cells – associated with intra-ocular infection (often postoperative) or severe corneal infective ulceration (Figs 2.15b, 2.33).

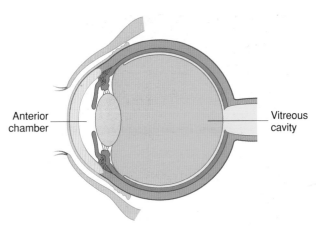

Anterior
chamber

Vitreous
cavity

Fig. 2.13b

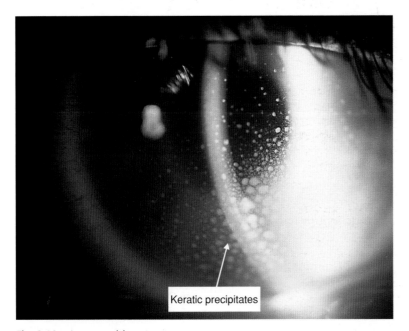

Keratic precipitates

Fig. 2.14   Acute uveitis.

Lens
A partial or total cataract may be associated with a penetrating injury if the
history is suggestive.

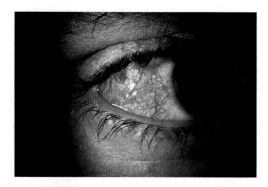

Fig. 2.15a Scleral injection – mild in episcleritis, severe in scleritis.

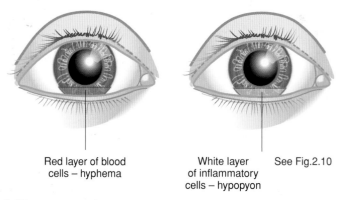

Red layer of blood cells – hyphema

White layer of inflammatory cells – hypopyon

See Fig.2.10

Fig. 2.15b

Fundus

Often difficult to examine adequately in acute cases – and rarely any pathology to account for an acute red eye.

General Examination

Not generally required but associations include:

- trauma – look for other injury if suspected
- connective tissue disorders – such as rheumatoid arthritis – may lead to dry eyes and corneal ulcers
- sarcoid – uveitis.

CORNEAL ABRASION (Figs 2.16, 2.17, 2.18a,b)

- acutely painful

- usually caused by a child's fingernail, gardening, mascara brushes, and after excess alcohol, when inadequate lid closure during sleep leads to corneal contact with bed linen
- can be recurrent.

Examination and Management

1. Instill a drop of combined topical anesthetic and fluorescein such as proxymetacaine 0.5% and fluorescein 0.25% to allow examination – separate preparations can be used.
2. Document visual acuity.

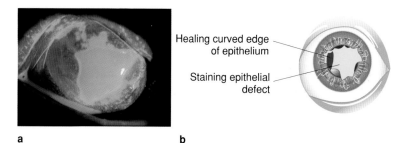

Healing curved edge of epithelium

Staining epithelial defect

a   b

Figs 2.16a,b Large corneal abrasion highlighted with fluorescein.

Linear scratches from foreign body under the eyelid - subtarsal foreign body

Figs 2.17 Linear abrasions from a subtarsal foreign body (see also Fig. 2.12).

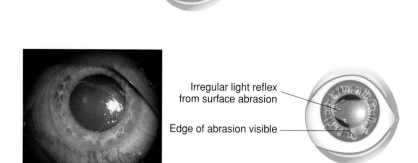

Irregular light reflex from surface abrasion

Edge of abrasion visible

a   b

Fig. 2.18a,b Corneal abrasion. Visible without fluorescein. Note irregular light reflex.

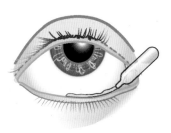
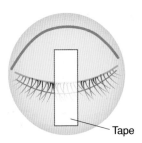

1 Ask patient to look up
Pull down lower lid
Instill chloramphenicol ointment
into lower fornix (gutter between
eye and eyelid)

2 Close eye
Tape lid down if necessary

Tape

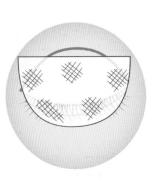
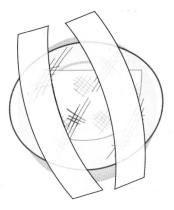

3 Fold eye patch in half and place
over closed lids

4 Cover with another patch
and tape down

Fig. 2.18c   Technique for double patching (Figs 9.13, 9.14, p. 158).

3. Abraded cornea appears green with fluorescein staining under a cobalt blue light – and is often easily visible with white light.
4. Look for a corneal foreign body – linear abrasions in the upper part of the cornea indicate a subtarsal foreign body (Fig. 2.12), and the upper lid should be everted in all cases (see p. 32).
5. Remove any foreign bodies; subtarsal particles can be removed with a cotton bud, corneal foreign bodies may require removal with a needle (see p. 29).
6. Relieve pain secondary to iris spasm with topical cyclopentolate 1% twice daily for 2 days.
7. Instill chloramphenicol ointment 1%.
8. Patch the eye with two eye pads as shown in Fig. 2.18c.

Double Eye Patch
- fold one patch in half and place over the closed eye
- place the other patch on top and tape down firmly
- ensure patient cannot easily open eye under patch – tape upper lid down if required.

1. Leave patches on undisturbed for 24 hours – they may not speed healing but patients are usually more comfortable with them.
2. Discharge on chloramphenicol 1% ointment four times daily for 5 days, starting after 24 hours.
3. Advise patient that the eye will become painful once the local anesthetic has worn off – usually within half an hour – they should not drive.
4. Simple oral analgesia as required.
5. Complete healing usually occurs within 48 hours.

To Instill Ointment

- patient should stand in front of a mirror
- pull down lower lid and squeeze a short line of ointment into the gutter formed between the inner surface of the lower lid and the eye
- ensure tube nozzle does not touch eye
- reassure that whilst most comes out on blinking sufficient is retained for therapeutic effect.

Infants

- may need to be wrapped in a blanket to restrain limbs and allow examination
- look for subtarsal (under the upper eyelid) foreign bodies – often difficult to do
- do not patch – child will simply pull it off
- always discuss with ophthalmologist.

Referral and Follow Up

- large (over 30% of corneal surface) abrasions, bilateral cases and children – discuss with the ophthalmologist
- all others review after 24 hours.

Pitfalls

- failure to examine for subtarsal foreign bodies.

CORNEAL FOREIGN BODY (Figs 2.19, 2.20, 2.21)

Features

- metallic corneal foreign bodies (FB) are common in industrial workers involved in drilling, grinding or welding

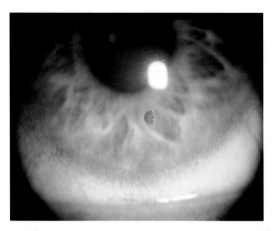

Fig. 2.19 Metallic foreign body – superficial with no rust ring at this early stage.

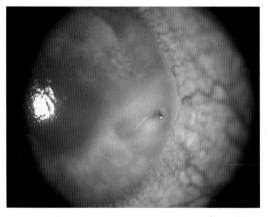

Fig. 2.20 Penetrating foreign body – note hazy cornea with irregular light reflex.

- dried paint FBs may be found in painters and decorators, and organic FBs in gardeners
- a subtarsal (under the upper lid) FB may coexist
- *both* eyes may have FBs.

Management

1. Instill a drop of combined topical anesthetic and fluorescein such as proxymetacaine 0.5% and fluorescein 0.25% to allow examination – separate preparations can be used.

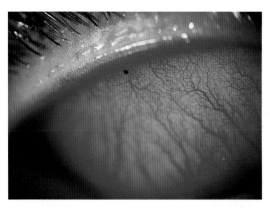

Fig. 2.21 Subtarsal foreign body – look for these even if you have already found a particle on the corneal surface as both may be present in the same eye.

2. Attempt to remove FB with a cotton bud – use a slit lamp if available or a magnifying loupe.
3. If you cannot remove the FB with a cotton bud, try to dislodge it with an orange needle (Fig. 2.24).

To Remove a Corneal FB Using a Needle (Figs 2.22–2.24)

1. Mount the needle on a 2 ml syringe which acts as a handle and gives you greater control.
2. Inform the patient what you are about to do, and reassure him that the needle 'does not go into the eye'.
3. Hold the upper eyelid to prevent blinking – to do this:
   - make them look down
   - place your thumb on the lower border of the upper lid and elevate the lid
   - ask the patient to look straight ahead, or whichever direction gives best access to the foreign body.
4. Gently try to remove the FB with the tip of the needle at a glancing (shallow) angle to the corneal surface – bend the needle if required as shown below.
5. Once the FB is dislodged pick it up with a damp cotton bud as this is easier than attempting to remove it from the surface of the eye with the needle
   - if a dense rust ring remains around the FB site after removal attempt to remove this as well – however it is often easier to remove 24 to 48 hours later
   - instill one drop of cyclopentolate 1% (Mydrilate 1%)
   - instill chloramphenicol ointment 1%
   - pad the eye with two eye pads for 24 hours (see Fig. 2.18c).

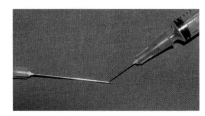

Fig. 2.22   Place tip of orange needle into the bore of a green needle and bend about 30 degrees – this produces a useful 'barb' to manipulate off a corneal foreign body.

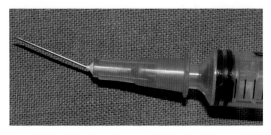

Fig. 2.23   Then bend the shaft about 30 degrees – this allows an easier tangential approach to the corneal surface.

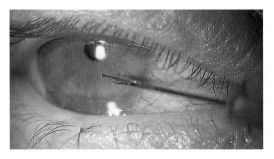

Fig. 2.24   Hold the eyelids and remove – top up local anesthetic if required.

Double Eye Pad
- fold one patch in half and place over the closed eye
- place the other patch on top and tape down firmly.

1. Discharge on chloramphenicol ointment 1% three times daily for 1 week.
2. Advise patient that pain will recur once the topical anesthetic wears off – usually within half an hour, but should settle within 24 hours.

Referral and Follow Up

- children – discuss with ophthalmologist immediately

- adults – ophthalmologist within 24 hours if you cannot completely remove the FB
- discharge all others.

Pitfalls

Failure to

- inquire about and search for possible penetrating injury
- examine other eye for foreign body
- look for subtarsal foreign bodies.

SUBTARSAL FOREIGN BODY (STFB)

Features

- no surface corneal foreign body usually seen
- patient often accurately describes 'something under the lid' and pain with blinking
- linear abrasions seen with fluorescein in the upper cornea are typical (Fig. 2.12).

Management

1. Instill a drop of proxymetacaine 0.5% topical anesthetic and stain with fluorescein.
2. Evert the upper lid over a cotton bud stick (Figs 2.25–2.28 and see Figs 2.17 and 2.21).
3. Remove the FB with a firm wipe from a cotton bud.
4. Drop of cyclopentolate 1% if photophobic (light is painful).
5. Chloramphenicol ointment 1%.
6. Pad with two eye pads for 24 hours if multiple abrasions are present.
7. Discharge on chloramphenicol ointment three times daily for 5 days.
8. Advise that pain will recur when the topical anesthetic wears off – usually in half an hour, but should settle within 24 hours.

Referral and Follow Up

- not required.

Pitfalls

Failure to

- inquire about and search for possible penetrating injury
- examine other eye for foreign body.

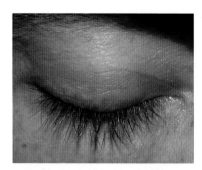

Fig. 2.25 Ask patient to look down and to keep looking down.

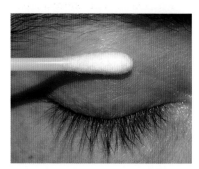

Fig. 2.26 Place a cotton bud gently on upper lid as shown.

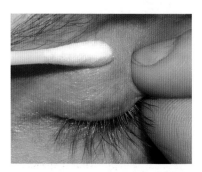

Fig. 2.27 Hold lashes firmly and rotate lid over cotton bud.

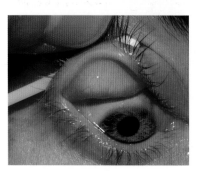

Fig. 2.28 Hold in place. The lid will flick back if the patient does not continue to look down.

INGROWING LASHES (TRICHIASIS) (Fig. 2.29); ENTROPION (Fig. 2.30a,b)

Features

■ trichiasis – inwardly directed lashes leading to abrasions
■ common and recurrent foreign body sensation
■ may affect both lower and upper lid
■ common usually in elderly.

Management

1. Differentiate between ingrowing or aberrant lashes and entropion (see above).
2. Stain the cornea with dilute fluorescein and look for lash-induced abrasions.

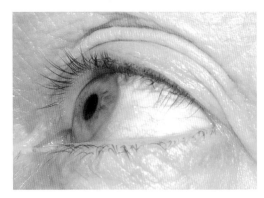

Fig. 2.29 Ingrowing eyelashes – affecting the upper lid temporally.

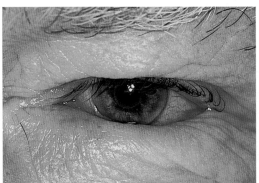

Fig. 2.30a Entropion – the whole lower lid has rolled in towards the eye. The lashes abrade both the cornea and conjunctiva.

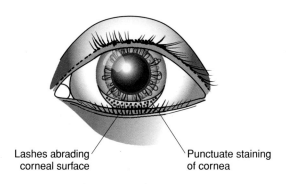

Lashes abrading corneal surface

Punctuate staining of cornea

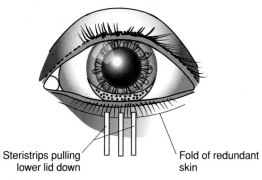

Steristrips pulling lower lid down

Fold of redundant skin

Fig. 2.30b Entropion – Steristrips or tape are a useful temporary measure.

3. If no entropion is present identify and epilate (pull out) the offending lashes.
4. If entropion is present – use Steristrips to pull the lower lid off the globe (Fig. 2.30b)
   - dry the skin
   - place one end of a Steristrip on the skin just below the lashes
   - pull down gently until lashes are pulled off the globe
   - stick other end onto cheek
   - use three Steristrips in a row.
5. If corneal staining is present, instill and disharge on chloramphenicol ointment 1% three times daily for 5 days.

Referral and Follow Up

- trichiasis and entropion – routine ophthalmology outpatient appointment
- if evidence of ocular infection – discuss with the ophthalmologist.

UVEITIS

Features

- photophobia (light is painful)
- perilimbal (junction between the cornea and sclera) injection
- small pupil and ocular tenderness
- often history of recurrence, particularly in young men with ankylosing spondylitis.

1. Listen to the patient if they state that this is a recurrent problem – they are usually well versed in the appropriate management.
2. Ensure that the patient does not have a corneal dendritic ulcer (Fig. 2.36).
3. If the uveitis is mild and the patient is not distressed, treat with:
   - steroid drops such as Pred Forte, Maxidex or Betnesol 2 hourly (**only start steroids if you are confident of the diagnosis and there is no history of cold sores or corneal ulcers**)
   - cyclopentolate (Mydrilate) 1% drops twice daily.
4. Check that the pupil dilates with this, if not it may be stuck to the lens (posterior synechiae) and stronger dilating agents are required, such as atropine 1% – discuss with the ophthalmologist.
5. Attempt to look at the fundus – uveitis may occur following retinal detachment or be secondary to an intraocular tumor.

Referral and Follow Up

- mild cases, patient not distressed – ophthalmologist within 24 hours
- severe cases – discuss immediately.

Pitfalls

- often mistreated as conjunctivitis – photophobia and pain are common in uveitis but rare in conjunctivitis
- recurrent or non-responding uveitis may be secondary to an intraocular tumor.

CONTACT LENS OVERWEAR

Features

- common – usually occurs as a result of failing to remove contact lenses before sleeping
- usually in soft or disposable lens wearers.

Management

1. Confirm that contact lenses have been removed.
2. Stain the cornea with fluorescein and observe under a blue light – a diffuse pattern of staining is common on the cornea centrally.

3. Ensure there is no corneal ulcer (see p. 38).
4. Cyclopentolate 1% stat.
5. Chloramphenicol ointment 1% stat.
6. Patch the eye – or the worst eye if both eyes involved with a double patch for 24 hours.

Double Eye Patch (Fig. 2.18c)
■ fold one patch in half and place over the closed eye
■ place the other patch on top and tape down firmly.

1. Discharge on chloramphenicol ointment 1% four times daily for 1 week.
2. Advise patient to leave out contact lenses during treatment.

Referral and Follow Up

■ review after 24 hours if not settling
■ optician once settled for contact lens check.

LOST CONTACT LENS (Fig. 2.31)

Features

■ may occur spontaneously or following trauma – typically sports related
■ often difficult to see with naked eye.

Management

1. Ensure that the patient has not already removed the lens.

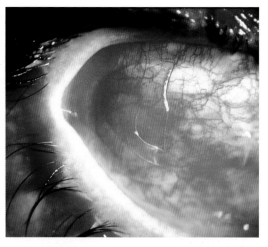

Fig. 2.31 This broken lens could also be subtarsal (under the upper lid) or tucked in the lower conjunctival fornix.

2. Instill topical anesthetic such as proxymetacaine 0.5%, benoxinate 0.4% or amethocaine 1%.
3. Use a slit lamp if available.
4. Examine the lower conjunctival fornix by (Fig. 2.32):
   - making the patient look up while you pull their lower lid down
   - ask them to look left and right whilst looking up
   - look for the lens in the folds of conjunctiva.
5. Evert the upper lid – to do this (see p. 32):
   - ask the patient to look down and keep looking down
   - place the wooden stick of a cotton bud horizontally across the mid portion of the upper lid – grasp their eyelashes firmly and gently rotate the lid upwards over the stick
   - ensure that they are still looking down – you cannot evert otherwise
   - remove the stick and hold the eyelid in position by holding the lashes
   - make the patient look left and right again to see if lens is exposed
   - if lens not found, sweep the cotton bud under the upper lid – uncomfortable.
6. If the lens is still not found instill fluorescein to highlight the lens and observe under a blue light repeating steps 3 & 4 – advise the patient that this will stain soft lenses.
7. If the lens is found ensure that it is intact – if part missing search for this.
8. Discharge on chloramphenicol ointment 1% four times daily for 5 days and advise patient not to re-insert lens for this period.
9. Patch the eye for 24 hours if abrasions are present.

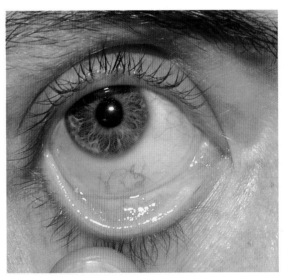

Fig. 2.32 Make sure you examine the lower conjunctival fornix as well as everting the upper lid.

Referral and Follow Up

- only required if lens is not found or part is missing – ophthalmologist within 24 hours
- all others to optician for check of lens fitting.

CORNEAL ULCER

Features

There are three main groups (Figs 2.33–2.36)

- **bacterial ulcers** – associated with contact lens wear and surface pathology such as dry eyes, or previous trauma – dense, usually bacterial but occasionally herpetic, often oval-shaped white opacity (Fig. 2.33)
- **ulcers associated with eyelid disease** – blepharitis and rosacea (ruddy cheeks and nose) may lead to ulcers at edge of cornea, often crescent shaped (marginal ulcer), related to exotoxins rather than frank infection (Figs 2.34, 2.35)
- **dendritic ulcers** – herpes virus, branching shape, may be single or multiple (Fig. 2.36).

Management

1. Differentiate type of ulcer according to history and features as above.

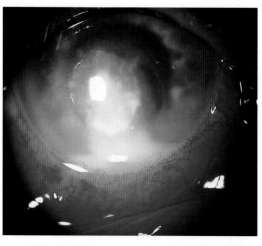

Fig. 2.33 Dense white deep ulcer and corneal abscess – note hypopyon (pus cell layer) in anterior chamber of eye.

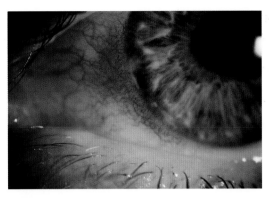

Fig. 2.34 Marginal ulcer – at the edge of the cornea.

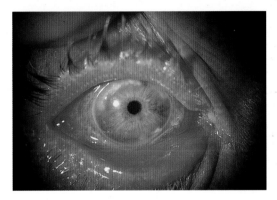

Fig. 2.35 Severe marginal ulceration – associated with severe blepharitis.

2. Instill a drop of fluorescein and observe under a blue light – this highlights an epithelial defect and makes superficial dendritic ulcers apparent.
3. Treat as below.

Contact-lens-related Ulcers

1. Should be seen by ophthalmologist the same day, if this is not possible within 24 hours, continue as below.
2. Scrape the ulcer with a sterile scalpel blade and plate for bacteriology – if you are not confident with this procedure, firmly swab with a sterile bud.
3. Take a viral swab.
4. Cefuroxime drops 5% hourly (50 mg/ml – you can mix this up from an IV preparation).

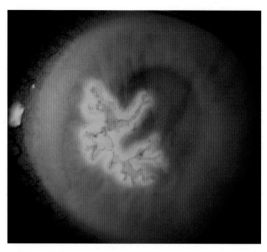

Fig. 2.36   Dendritic ulcer – typical shape.

5. Genticin drops 1.5% hourly (add 4 ml sterile water to 80 mg/2 ml phial of IV Genticin).
6. Atropine 1% drops three times daily.

Dendritic Ulcers

1. Zovirax ointment 3% five times a day for 5 days – ensure that this is the eye preparation and not for skin use.
2. Cyclopentolate 1% drops twice daily.
3. Small dendritic ulcer will usually resolve within 5–7 days on adequate treatment.

Marginal Ulcers

1. Chloramphenicol ointment four times daily for 1 week.
2. Cyclopentolate 1% drops twice daily if the eye is very painful.
3. These settle rapidly with topical steroids such as Predsol 0.5% three times daily for one week – let the ophthalmologist start this form of treatment unless you are confident of the diagnosis.
4. Treat blepharitis if present (see p. 143).

Referral and Follow Up

- **contact lens related** – ophthalmologist immediately
- **dendritic ulcer** – ophthalmologist within 24 hours for large ulcers – all others, review in 5 days and refer if not healed
- **marginal ulcer** – ophthalmologist within 24 hours
- **any other ulcer** – discuss with ophthalmologist immediately.

Pitfalls

- never start topical steroids without ophthalmological advice and close ophthalmological follow up
- do not delay treatment – bacterial ulcers can rapidly destroy an eye.

PENETRATING AND BLUNT INJURY

See Chapter 5 (trauma, p. 112).

ACUTE GLAUCOMA

Features

- predominantly elderly patients
- debilitated patient with intense ocular pain
- abdominal pain and vomiting may be present
- cornea may be cloudy, with a fixed semi-dilated pupil and vision markedly reduced
- the eye feels rock hard when palpated through the eyelid.

Management

1. Diamox 500 mg intravenously.
2. Pilocarpine 2% drops to both eyes – every hour to the affected eye, four times daily to the unaffected eye. This may have little effect initially until the Diamox reduces eye pressure.
3. Pred Forte, Maxidex or Betnesol one drop hourly to the affected eye.
4. Analgesia is very important and often forgotten – pethidine 50 mg or diamorphine 5 mg intramuscular – adjusted according to the weight of the patient.
5. Antiemetic – do not give by mouth – Stemetil (prochlorperazine) 12.5 mg intramuscular or Maxolon (metoclopramide) 10 mg intramuscular.

Referral and Follow Up

- admit immediately under the ophthalmologists.

EPISCLERITIS AND SCLERITIS (Figs 2.37, 2.38a,b)

Features

- may involve whole or just part of the sclera and usually unilateral
- scleritis is painful and may keep the patient awake at night
- episcleritis is either asymptomatic or mildly irritable.

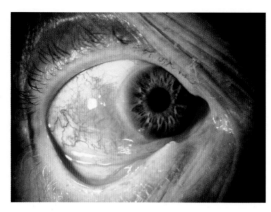

Fig. 2.37   Sector of inflammation is characteristic in episcleritis.

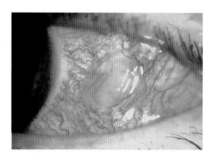

Fig. 2.38a   More severe episcleritis with conjunctival nodule.

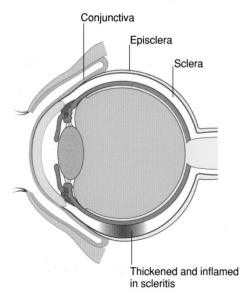

Conjunctiva

Episclera

Sclera

Thickened and inflamed in scleritis

Fig. 2.38b   Inflammation of the sclera is more serious and may result in severe pain in comparison with more superficial episcleritis.

Management

1. Document visual acuity which may be reduced in scleritis.
2. Stain with fluorescein to rule out an abrasion or foreign body – if present evert the lids and look for a subtarsal foreign body (see p. 32).
3. Look for ingrowing eyelashes or a lash in the lacrimal punctum if the injection is nasally situated.
4. Asymptomatic or mild irritation, probable diagnosis is episcleritis – no treatment required (Fig. 2.48).
5. If irritable, start on a non-steroidal anti-inflammatory agent such as Froben 100 mg twice daily by mouth with food – provided there are no contraindications – or Voltarol drops three times daily for 10 days.
6. Do not start on topical steroids unless early follow up with ophthalmologist is possible.

Referral and Follow Up

- acute pain – discuss immediately with the ophthalmologist – high-dose intravenous steroids may be required as an inpatient
- minor symptoms – treat as above for 10 days and review at 2 weeks
- asymptomatic – reassure and discharge.

Pitfalls

- non-steroidal anti-inflammatory agents may lead to severe gastro-intestinal symptoms – warn the patient to stop treatment and return should this occur
- a lash in the lacrimal punctum may mimic the condition – look carefully for this.

SHINGLES (Figs 2.39, 2.40, 8.7)

Features

- shingles affecting the ophthalmic division of the trigeminal nerve or herpes zoster ophthalmicus (HZO) accounts for 10% of shingles
- skin distribution is characteristic, may be barely apparent or severe and can lead to lid scarring with entropion and trichiasis (see p. 151)
- eye involvement includes corneal micro-ulcers, uveitis, glaucoma and optic neuritis.

Management

1. Document visual acuity in each eye using a pinhole if required (see p. 5).
2. Stain the cornea with fluorescein and look for ulceration (see p. 38).
3. Examine the anterior chamber for flare or cells indicating uveitis (see p. 35).

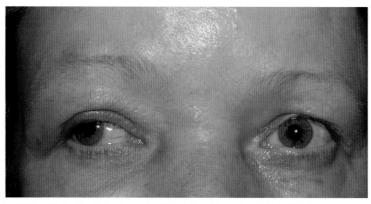

Fig. 2.39 Note the lid edema on the right side – the other skin features are very subtle in this early stage – once vesicles are seen the diagnosis is straightforward – this patient also has a right divergent squint.

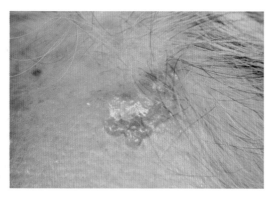

Fig. 2.40 Vesicles in herpes zoster – look in the hairline and scalp.

4. Treat uveitis with topical Betnesol or Pred Forte 4× daily and cyclopentolate 1% 2× daily.
5. Intraocular pressure is often raised secondary to uveitis – add topical beta blocker such as Timoptol 0.5% 2× daily or if contraindicated (asthmatic) topical latanoprost (Xalatan) one drop daily.
6. If only the eyelids are involved but the eye is quiet, you do not need to treat as above (refer to p. 149; Lids – shingles).
7. Zovirax shingles pack (800 mg 5× day for 1 week orally).
8. Zovirax eye ointment is not required.
9. Analgesia – oral or intramuscular as pain secondary to neuralgia can be excruciating – amitryptyline is sometimes effective – 25 mg once daily by month as a starting dose (beware of urinary retention and cardiotoxicity).

Referral and Follow Up

- eye and lid involvement – ophthalmologist within 24 hours
- lid involvement only – review in 3 days
- advise patient to return immediately if new eye symptoms develop.

RED EYE – ACUTE, PAINFUL, BILATERAL

Common Causes

chemical injury – alkali or acid	p. 112 – **wash out eyes now**
welding/grinding	p. 48
trauma – blunt or sharp	p. 114, 125
contact lens wear	p. 49

Consider

dry eyes	p. 63
conjunctivitis	p. 51
allergic reaction	p. 50
dysthyroid eye disease	p. 53
carotico-cavernous fistula	p. 54

Ask Directly

- **chemical splashed into the eye. Wash out now** – with copious amounts of water or saline before any further questions or examination (see p. 112)
- **welding or grinding.** Welders flash from UV light occurs if goggles are not worn – grinding may lead to bilateral corneal foreign bodies (see p. 27)
- **dry eyes.** Very common, more frequent in elderly and those with connective tissue disease – usually chronic
- **contact lenses.** Contact lens overwear (usually due to sleeping with lenses in) and failure to adequately rinse them after using cleaning solution is common
- **discharge from eye.** Conjunctivitis is usually just irritable – some viral infections however may be painful
- **sore, itchy eyelids.** Blepharitis (see p. 143) is common, often presents as sore, red eyes and may be associated with corneal ulcers (see p. 38)
- **eye drop allergy.** Allergy to antibiotic drops may be associated with excoriated skin and lid swelling (Fig. 2.41)
- **recent flu or cold.** Viral keratoconjunctivitis may follow upper respiratory tract viral infection
- **thyroid disease.** Consider thyroid eye disease which may present with conjunctival chemosis, erythema and discomfort and can occur in a euthyroid patient

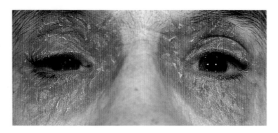

Fig. 2.41   Allergy to eye drops – severe periorbital skin excoriation may occur.

■ **head injury.** Carotico-cavernous fistula is extremely rare and may be secondary to trauma, or spontaneous in elderly hypertensives.

Examination

External
1. Look for signs of trauma – particularly chemical burns to the face.
2. Proptotic, bulging eyes, staring expression – thyroid disease (Fig. 2.42a).

Visual Acuity
1. Reduced from watering and blepharospasm (eyes tightly closed) quite apart from other pathology.
2. Instill a drop of proxymetacaine 0.5%, benoxinate 0.4% or amethocaine 1% if blepharospasm is present – this may relieve discomfort and allow further examination.
3. Conjunctivitis rarely leads to significantly reduced vision whereas thyroid eye disease may lead to severe visual loss from corneal exposure or optic nerve compression.

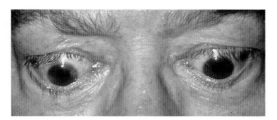

Fig. 2.42a   Dysthyroid eye disease – note upper lid retraction.

Fig. 2.42b   Red target – use this to check colour vision.

Color Perception
1. If a red object appears less red or a light less bright in one eye compared with the other then consider optic nerve compression – particularly thyroid eye disease (see p. 53) or orbital cellulitis (Fig. 8.4a,b)
2. Check color vision in each eye individually – use the red spot shown in Fig. 2.42b.

Fields
1. Unnecessary to check visual fields (see p. 10) in primary care setting unless patient complains of field loss or neurological defect suspected.

Pupils
1. May be small due to inflammation or enlarged following trauma – a blunt injury can damage the iris sphincter muscle.
2. An afferent pupil defect (see p. 7) indicates optic nerve dysfunction, requires urgent referral and if in the presence of an orbital hematoma following trauma, decompression (see p. 122).

Lids
1. Crusting and erythema around the eyelashes indicate blepharitis – look for associated corneal ulcers (see p. 38).
2. Usually a long history of ocular and lid irritation prior to the acute episode of blepharitis.

Conjunctiva
1. Injection may be secondary to corneal or intraocular pathology rather than simply conjunctivitis.
2. Instill fluorescein drop and look for abrasions on the conjunctiva as well as the cornea.
3. Chemical injury may lead to diffuse staining if mild, or gross loss of conjunctival and corneal epithelium – severe cases may show white areas of 'normal' looking tissue – due to complete destruction of vascular tissue.
4. Markedly swollen conjunctiva in the absence of trauma may be secondary to allergy or thyroid eye disease.

Cornea
1. Stain with fluorescein and look for surface and subtarsal foreign bodies (see p. 27, 31).
2. Diffuse staining occurs in mild chemical injury, viral kerato-conjunctivitis, contact lens and UV light (welding flash) injuries.
3. Gross epithelial loss may occur in chemical injury.
4. Bilateral simultaneous dendritic ulcers are rare.

Sclera
1. Difficult to differentiate between conjunctival, episcleral and scleral injection.
2. Severe pain and injection indicates scleritis (see p. 41) – but this is rare bilaterally.
3. Visual acuity is often reduced in scleritis.

Anterior Chamber
1. Look for signs of inflammation – injection around the cornea and photophobia indicate uveitis (Fig. 2.6).
2. Bilateral acute uveitis is uncommon and rarely leads to a red eye.
3. Bilateral simultaneous acute glaucoma is extremely unlikely.

Fundus
1. Usually little to see – vitreous debris can occur in uveitis – the patient may see these as floaters (Figs 4.10b, 4.22).

General Examination
1. Look for other sites of injury in chemical or other trauma and treat appropriately.
2. Examine for signs of hyperthyroidism (see p. 53).

Pitfalls
- bilateral conjunctival chemosis in dysthyroid eye disease may be attributed to conjunctivitis or an allergic response
- optic nerve compression resulting in an afferent pupil defect (see p. 7) can lead to permanent visual loss if not promptly and appropriately treated.

WELDING, GRINDING AND FLASH BURN INJURIES

Features
- commonly bilateral and recurrent.

Management
1. Instill topical anesthetic such as proxymetacaine 0.5%, benoxinate 0.4% or amethocaine 1.0% to allow examination.
2. Instill fluorescein and look under a blue light for abrasions and foreign bodies (FB) (see p. 27).
3. Remove FB if present and treat as an abrasion (see p. 24).
4. Cyclopentolate 1% to both eyes.
5. Chloramphenicol ointment 1% into both eyes.
6. Patch worst eye for 24 hours.
7. Discharge on chloramphenicol ointment four times daily for 5 days.

Referral and Follow Up

- if FB cannot be removed treat as above and refer to ophthalmologist within 24 hours
- unnecessary if FB removed easily.

Pitfalls

- do not overlook the potential for a penetrating injury (see p. 125)
- failure to X-ray the orbit if the history includes hammering or chiselling – look for evidence of a penetrating injury or intraocular foreign body (Fig. 5.17a).

CONTACT LENS WEAR RELATED

Features

- usually related to overwear or failure to rinse adequately after chemically cleaning
- acute allergic response to soft lenses may occur after many trouble-free years.

Management

1. Ensure contact lenses have been removed – use topical anesthetic such as proxymetacaine 0.5%, benoxinate 0.4% or amethocaine 1.0% to allow examination if required.
2. Fluorescein will stain soft lenses – advise patient, and use to help locate lens if lost (see p. 36).
3. Once lenses have been removed look for abrasions, ulcers, or diffuse staining indicating overwear (often as a result of sleeping with lenses in) or chemical injury due to lens cleaning solution.
4. Irrigate if history implicates contact lens cleaning solution.
5. In severe cases instill a drop of cyclopentolate 1% to relieve ciliary muscle spasm and pain.
6. Chloramphenicol ointment 1% into affected eye(s).
7. Treat diffuse staining as an abrasion (see p. 24) and patch the worst eye.
8. If an ulcer is present (see p. 38) refer as below.
9. Discharge on chloramphenicol ointment 1% four times daily for 5 days.
10. Instruct patient to leave out contact lenses until they have been checked for foreign bodies by their optician and not to re-insert them for a minimum of 1 week.

Referral and Follow Up

- corneal ulcer – discuss with ophthalmologist immediately

- punctate staining – review within 24 hours – if not improving discuss with ophthalmologist
- advise patient to see optician as in 10 above.

ALLERGIC REACTION TO EYE DROPS OR CONTACT LENSES

Features

- typically from antibiotic eye drops started for conjunctivitis
- periorbital skin may be excoriated, erythematous and edematous (Fig. 2.41).

Management

1. Identify any drops recently started – usually for conjunctivitis.
2. Remove contact lenses if in situ using topical anesthesia if required such as proxymetacaine 0.5%, benoxinate 0.4% or amethocaine 1.0%.
3. Stop any new antibiotic drops and change to an alternative if required – common antibiotic drops include chloramphenicol, Genticin, Exocin and Fucithalmic – neomycin is often used in combination with a steroid (Betnesol-N).
4. Glaucoma drops should not be stopped unless discussed with the ophthalmologist
   - atropine, Propine, Alphagan – reaction not uncommon
   - Betoptic, Timoptol, Xalatan, pilocarpine – reaction less common.
5. Cold compresses over both eyes improves comfort and reduces swelling.
6. Contact lenses should not be replaced until reviewed by ophthalmologist.
7. If fluid-filled clear conjunctiva – often with edema of surrounding skin (Fig. 8.2)
   - probable response to allergen such as pollen or house dust
   - usually acute onset within one or two hours
   - responds to ice packs over closed eyes
   - Otrivine, Rapitil or Opatanol drops four times daily until settled
   - oral antihistamines.

Referral and Follow Up

- review next day
- ophthalmologist within 24 hours if fails to respond to above treatment.

CONJUNCTIVITIS (Fig. 2.43)

Features

- rarely leads to a painful eye unless the cornea is also involved as in viral keratoconjunctivitis
- patients may complain of pain which on questioning is simply irritation
- discharge indicates bacterial conjunctivitis whereas excess lacrimation (watering) is associated with viral infections.

Management

1. Look for discharge in tear film – easily seen with slit lamp.
2. Stain with fluorescein and look for characteristic punctate staining of adenovirus.
3. Follicles – pale pink gelatinous-looking globules within the conjunctiva indicate viral disease – if associated with a discharge in sexually active individuals consider chlamydia and take swabs.
4. Chloramphenicol drops 1% four times daily to both eyes for 10 days.
5. If chlamydia suspected treat with tetracycline ointment 1% and oral tetracycline 250 mg, both four times daily for 3 weeks – sexual partners also require treatment.

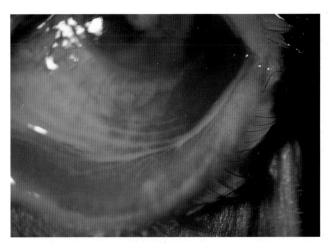

Fig. 2.43 Conjunctivitis with discharge. Reproduced with permission from Kanski J J, 2003, Clinical Ophthalmology: A Systemic Approach, Butterworth-Heinemann.

6. If patient has already been treated with no effect (first-line therapy is usually chloramphenicol) take a conjunctival swab by asking the patient to look up and sweeping the lower conjunctival fornix with the swab.
7. Treat with an alternative antibiotic in the case of bacterial conjunctivitis such as fusidic acid 1% (Fucithalmic) ointment twice daily, Ciloxan, Exocin or gentamicin (Genticin) four times daily.

Referral and Follow Up

■ visual loss or severe pain – discuss with the ophthalmologist and refer within 24 hours
■ not required in routine cases unless symptoms do not improve or worsen over 3–4 days
■ suspected chlamydia should be reviewed in ophthalmology outpatients after 1–2 weeks of treatment.

VIRAL KERATOCONJUNCTIVITIS

Features

■ commonly associated with upper respiratory tract infection
■ often contact with similarly affected individuals
■ usual organism is an adenovirus
■ bilateral dendritic ulceration can occur if immunosuppressed.

Management

1. Instill topical anesthesia such as proxymetacaine 0.5% , benoxinate 0.4% or amethocaine 1.0% if the patient is unable to open their eyes.
2. Stain the cornea with fluorescein.
3. Adenovirus stains lightly as multiple punctate spots best seen under the slit lamp – dendritic ulcers have a characteristic branching pattern (Fig. 2.36).
4. If adenovirus suspected discharge on chloramphenicol drops four times daily to each eye to prevent secondary infection for 2 weeks.
5. In severe cases add cyclopentolate 1% (Mydrilate) twice daily – warn the patient may blur vision.
6. Topical lubricants such as GelTears or Viscotears may be used for comfort.
7. Steroid drops are often required – leave this to the ophthalmologist.
8. If dendritic ulcers are present treat with Zovirax ointment 3% five times daily (see p. 40).

Wash your hands thoroughly – adenovirus is extremely contagious and easily spreads to health care workers.

Referral and Follow Up

■ ophthalmology outpatients within 1 week
■ adenovirus has a naturally resolving course but may last for months – advise the patient
■ bilateral dendritic ulcers are rare and should be reviewed by the ophthalmologist within 48 hours – suspect immunosuppression.

DYSTHYROID EYE DISEASE (Figs 2.44, 2.45)

Features

■ may occur in a euthyroid patient
■ sight-threatening complications from corneal exposure secondary to exophthalmos or optic nerve compression secondary to increased orbital pressure
■ gross chemosis (swelling and edema of the conjunctiva) may be present
■ diplopia, lid retraction, reduced acuity and eye movements common.

Management

1. Document visual acuity in each eye with glasses or pinhole if required (see p. 5).
2. An afferent pupil defect (see p. 7) indicates compression of the optic nerve and must be referred immediately.
3. If a long delay in obtaining an ophthalmology opinion is anticipated in the presence of pupil dysfunction start on high-dose parenteral

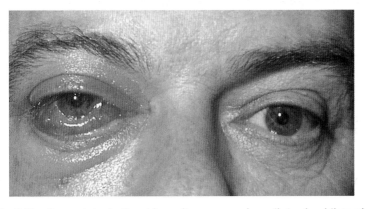

Fig. 2.44 Chemosis in dysthyroid eye disease – may be unilateral or bilateral and often treated as a non-resolving conjunctivitis.

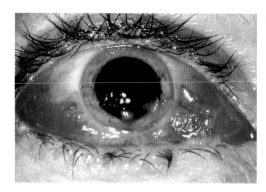

Fig. 2.45 Dysthyroid eye disease – severe conjunctival chemosis with corneal exposure – this patient also had optic nerve compression.

steroids – up to 1.5 g methylprednisolone intravenously depending upon weight.

4. 80 mg oral prednisolone enteric coated in conjunction with ranitidine 150 mg or lansoprazole (Zoton) 30 mg twice daily if unable to admit for parenteral therapy.

5. Usual precautions with high-dose steroids in those with a history of peptic ulceration or hypertension.

6. Fluorescein staining of cornea indicates exposure – treat with Lacri-Lube ointment four times daily and advise patient to tape down upper eyelids at night with a thin sliver of tape.

Referral and Follow Up

- reduced vision, pupil defect or corneal staining – immediate referral to ophthalmologist
- no signs of corneal exposure or optic nerve dysfunction – review by the ophthalmologist within 48 hours.

Pitfall

- thyroid conjunctival chemosis may be treated inappropriately as conjunctivitis – there is no discharge in dysthyroid eye disease.

CAROTICO-CAVERNOUS FISTULA

Features

- rare and dramatic condition from fistula between internal carotid and cavernous sinus
- bilateral conjunctival edema and pulsatile exophthalmos as venous outflow is compromised by arterial inflow
- spontaneous in elderly secondary to arteriosclerosis or following trauma in the young.

Referral and Follow Up

■ discuss immediately with neurosurgeons who will organize ophthalmology opinion if required.

RED EYE – ACUTE, PAINLESS, UNILATERAL

Main Causes

conjunctivitis	p. 56
subconjunctival hemorrhage	p. 57
episcleritis	p. 58
allergic reaction	p. 50

Ask Directly

■ **any discharge.** Yellow or white discharge common in bacterial conjunctivitis – watery discharge may occur in viral or an incompletely treated bacterial conjunctivitis

■ **history of any Valsalva maneuver or trauma** – for instance carrying heavy weights coughing or sneezing fits. Subconjunctival hemorrhage common following sudden increase in venous pressure

■ **hypertension or diabetes.** Spontaneous subconjunctival hemorrhage more common in these groups

■ **previous episodes.** Recurrence is common in all of the above conditions.

Examination

External
1. Ensure that there is no swelling of the lids or periorbital tissue which would indicate orbital cellulitis (see p. 147).

Visual Acuity
1. Usually unaffected in all of the above conditions although minimal reduction with severe conjunctivitis can occur.

Conjunctiva
1. Discharge indicates bacterial conjunctivitis.
2. Solid area of redness typical of subconjunctival hemorrhage

■ identify and document whether the upper edge of the hemorrhage is visible

■ if not, blood may have tracked forwards from an intracranial source – although this is extremely rare and usually follows head injury or subarachnoid hemorrhage

■ appearance may be alarming with the conjunctiva prolapsing over the lower lid (similar to Fig. 2.44).

Sclera

1. Segmental area of inflammation over the 'white' of the eye indicates episcleritis (Fig. 2.48) – this is an inflammation of the superficial layer of the sclera – features include:
   - no discharge
   - slight irritation
   - frequent recurrence
   - diffuse episcleritis may mimic conjunctivitis but is not associated with a discharging or 'sticky' eye.

Cornea, Pupil and Fundus

Cornea, pupils and fundus are usually normal in the above conditions.

CONJUNCTIVITIS (Fig. 2.46)

Features

- discharge may be purulent or watery
- irritable rather than painful.

Management

1. Severe cases – take a bacterial swab – ask patient to look up, pull down lower lid and sweep lower conjunctival fornix.
2. Stain with fluorescein and examine cornea under blue light for corneal lesions, such as dendritic ulcer (see p. 40) or foreign body (see p. 27) as these may be relatively painless.
3. Discharge on chloramphenicol drops 1% 2 hourly for 2 days then four times for 8 days.
4. If already on treatment which has failed take swab and start alternative antibiotic drops – see p. 52.
5. Ensure that patient is using previous treatment and has done so for at least 3 days.

Referral and Follow Up

- no referral usually required

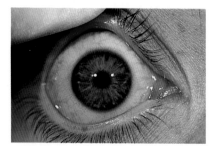

Fig. 2.46 Conjunctivitis – diffuse injection with purulent discharge. These may be subtle initially and uncomfortable or irritable rather than painful.

- ophthalmologist within 24 hours if treatment has failed after 5 days of adequate therapy or if pain or substantially reduced visual acuity are present.

SUBCONJUNCTIVAL HEMORRHAGE (Fig. 2.47)

Features

- usually spontaneous
- may be related to hypertension or following any Valsalva maneuver.

Management

1. Identify the upper border of the hemorrhage and document this.
2. Check blood pressure and treat if required.
3. Urinalysis for diabetes.
4. If no history of ocular or head trauma – reassure patient and advise that it will spontaneously resolve, but may take 6 weeks and can worsen before improvement.
5. No eye treatment is necessary.

Referral and Follow Up

- no referral required in spontaneous cases
- trauma related (examine as per Chapter 5)
- diabetes or hypertension – to GP or physicians as appropriate.

Pitfall

- identify and document that the upper border of the hemorrhage can be seen – make patient look down and lift the upper lid – if no

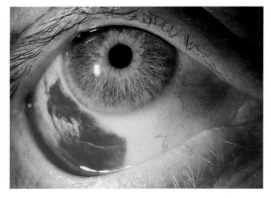

Fig. 2.47 Well-defined edge to hemorrhage – but may extend to cover most of sclera.

border is visible and the patient has a severe headache discuss with neurosurgeons – the blood may have tracked along the optic nerve from an intracranial source – however the patient is likely to be unwell if this is the case.

EPISCLERITIS (Fig. 2.48)

Features

- well defined sector of 'white' of eye involved – but may be diffuse
- irritation frequent.

Management

1. Stain with fluorescein and look for other lesions which cause a similar localized inflammation such as marginal corneal ulcer (Figs 2.34, 2.35) or corneal foreign body (see p. 27) – these may occasionally be painless.
2. If discomfort start on topical anti-inflammatory drops – Voltarol three times daily for one week. Froben 100 mg twice daily by mouth for 2 weeks may be used – provided no contraindications such as peptic ulceration or concomitant anti-inflammatory treatment.
3. Warn patient to stop treatment immediately and re-attend should any gastric irritation occur.
4. If recurrent in patient under 30 check renal function as episcleritis is a rare initial manifestation of renal failure in this age group.
5. Advise patient that condition usually resolves spontaneously in 2–3 weeks.

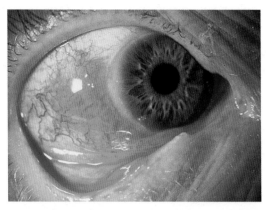

Fig. 2.48   Sector of inflammation with no hemorrhage – the yellow liquid is fluorescein dye.

Referral and Follow up

- not required – provided patient is off all treatment within 2 weeks
- ophthalmologist within 48 hours – if not settled on above treatment for 2 weeks as topical steroids may be required.

RED EYE – ACUTE, PAINLESS, BILATERAL

Main Causes

conjunctivitis	p. 56 (Fig. 2.46)
blepharitis – inflammation of the lid margins with secondary ocular irritation	p. 143
allergic reactions	p. 50
thyroid eye disease – rare	p. 53

Ask Directly

- **Discharge.** Mucopurulent discharge associated with bacterial conjunctivitis – consider chlamydia in the sexually active age group
- **Atopy.** Atopes are prone to allergic reactions from numerous allergens typically house dust or pollen
- **Known thyroid disease or symptoms or signs suggestive of hyperthyroidism.** Tremor, anxiety, temper, heat intolerance, palpitations, tachycardia or weight loss suggest thyroid overactivity – bilateral red eyes may be the initial presentation of thyroid disease, and may be inappropriately treated as conjunctivitis (see p. 53).

Examination

External
1. Swelling of the lids or periorbital tissues may indicate orbital cellulitis but this is rarely bilateral (see p. 147).

Visual Acuity
1. Usually unaffected in all of the above with exception of thyroid eye disease.
2. Minimal reduction common in severe conjunctivitis.

Conjunctiva
1. Discharge indicates bacterial conjunctivitis.
2. Pull down lower lid and look at the lower conjunctiva in the gutter between the eye and the inner part of the lower lid – grayish translucent globules (best seen under a slit lamp) are associated with chlamydial infection which should be suspected in the sexually active.
3. Evert upper lid (see p. 32) – a roughened injected undersurface occurs in atopic conjunctivitis.

Sclera
1. Injection over medial and lateral aspect of the sclera may indicate thyroid eye disease particularly if the eyes look prominent.

Cornea
1. Stain with fluorescein and look for an ulcer – diffuse staining may be related to exposure secondary to thyroid disease.
2. Marginal ulcers (see p. 40) are associated with blepharitis (see p. 143) – may present with mild discomfort rather than pain.

Pupils
1. An afferent pupillary defect (see p. 7) may indicate optic nerve compression secondary to thyroid disease.

Fundus
1. Fundal appearance is usually normal although small folds in the retina can occasionally be seen in thyroid disease.

CONJUNCTIVITIS

This is fully covered on page 51.

BLEPHARITIS (Figs 2.49, 2.50)

Features

- extremely common eyelid problem – leads to chronic bilateral ocular irritation rather than pain
- red crusty thickened lid margins
- acute exacerbations common
- eyelashes may be matted, crusted and have small flakes of adherent skin attached.

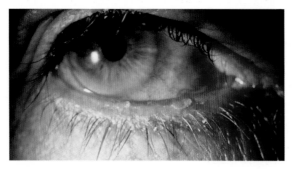

Fig. 2.49 Blepharitis. Thickened injected lid margins with discharge and crusting on lashes.

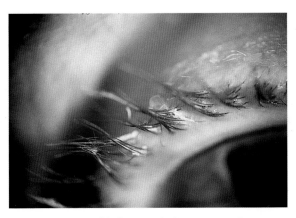

Fig. 2.50 Blepharitis. Matted lashes – typical appearance in severe cases.

Management

1. Advise patient that the condition is chronic and treatment is to relieve symptoms but will not cure the underlying problem.
2. Stain with fluorescein and look for corneal marginal ulcer (Figs 2.34, 2.35).
3. If lids are very injected start on chloramphenicol ointment 1% three times daily – this should be firmly rubbed into the eyelid margin at the base of the eyelashes for 3 weeks – there is no need to instill this into the eye.
4. Lid hygiene – advise the patient to clean the lid margins thoroughly morning and night by
   - pulling the skin of the outer lid margins laterally to put the lids under tension
   - with a clean lint cloth, cotton handkerchief or flannel dampened with a mild solution of saline (one teaspoon of salt in a tumbler of cooled boiled water) or baby shampoo – firmly rub the margins to remove grease and debris associated with the condition – but avoid touching the eye itself
   - continue treatment indefinitely
   - do not use cotton wool or cotton buds – these may leave debris in the eye.

Referral and Follow Up

- ophthalmologist within 48 hours if corneal staining is present
- not required in the absence of corneal pathology.

ALLERGIC REACTIONS

This is covered fully on page 50.

DYSTHYROID EYE DISEASE

This is fully covered on page 53.

RED EYE – CHRONIC, UNILATERAL OR BILATERAL

Main Causes

blepharitis	p. 60, 143
dry eye	p. 63
chronic conjunctivitis	p. 51
contact lens wear	p. 139
dysthyroid eye disease	p. 53
work (environment) related	

Ask Directly

- **Crusting or stuck down eyelids.** Typical of blepharitis
- **Arthritis.** Dry eye is common in the elderly, those on antidepressants and is also associated with rheumatoid arthritis
- **Contact lenses.** Lens intolerance and poor lens hygiene should be considered
- **Discharge.** Chronic conjunctivitis is a less common cause of chronic red eye
- **Work related.** Do they work in a dry dusty conditions or with air conditioning
- **History of thyroid disease.** Commonly treated as chronic conjunctivitis until properly diagnosed.

Examination

External
1. Look for the staring appearance associated with thyroid eye disease (see p. 53).

Lids
1. Red thickened lid margins with matted, crusty lashes (Fig. 2.50) that are matted together indicates blepharitis and occasionally a lid tumor, especially if lashes are absent.

Conjunctiva
1. Chronic alcohol abuse – suffused appearance.
2. Discharge – consider chronic conjunctivitis or chlamydia in the sexually active.
3. Rheumatoid arthritis – associated with dry eye common and leads to reduced tear film containing debris.

Cornea

1. Dry eyes lead to corneal exposure – and gritty sensation – stains diffusely with fluorescein.

Chronic red eye is usually due to external eye disease and further examination is unnecessary in the presence of normal visual acuity – if vision is reduced check the fundus for any gross abnormalities. Reduced vision is discussed on page 73.

Management

blepharitis	p. 60, 143
conjunctivitis	p. 51
thyroid eye disease	p. 53
contact lens problems	p. 35, 139

DRY EYE

Features

- chronic irritation with burning sensation
- diffuse injection.

Management

1. Stain with fluorescein and observe under a blue light – diffuse areas of fine punctate staining indicates dry eye.
2. Start on hypromellose 0.3% drops every 2 hours or Viscotears six times daily and Lacri-Lube ointment at night.

Referral and Follow Up

- corneal staining – ophthalmology outpatient appointment routinely once treatment started
- no corneal staining – no referral required.

Chapter 3

Painful Eye

Common complaint usually related to ocular trauma or inflammation. If the following features are present, go to relevant page

red eye   p. 113
trauma history   p. 112
reduced vision   p. 73
double vision   p. 107
intense pain with nausea   p. 41 (glaucoma)

PAINFUL EYE, NORMAL APPEARANCE, NORMAL VISION

■ common complaint with frequently no identifiable cause.

Consider

temporal arteritis	– elderly patient, headache	p. 74
sinusitis	– often a past history or recent cold	p. 67
neuralgia	– may follow ophthalmic shingles	p. 69
old glasses	– incorrect glasses may cause a headache	p. 71
migraine	– often a strong family history	p. 68
diabetes	– may be associated with a 6th, 3rd or 4th nerve palsy	p. 70
ischemia	– ocular ischemia often secondary to carotid disease	p. 71
optic neuritis	– an afferent pupil defect (see p. 7) is usually present	p. 88

Relevant Questions

1. **Is temporal arteritis a possibility?** Malaise, weight loss, jaw pain with eating (claudication), shoulder girdle pain, scalp tenderness, transient episodes of visual loss, age over 70 but can occur in 50s.
2. **Is the pain in the eye itself, or surrounding the eye?** Periocular pain is often described as 'eye' pain and may be referred from the temporomandibular joint, ear or sinuses. Reduced color vision associated with optic neuritis.

3. **Wearing old or inappropriate glasses, or having difficulty and pain when reading?** Incorrect glasses, or the need for spectacles, particularly in a middle-aged patient who experiences difficulty with reading is a common cause of visual discomfort.

4. **Is there a history of:**
   - **diabetes, hypertension, smoking.** All may lead to ocular ischemia and dull persistant periocular pain
   - **cold or sinusitis.** Sinusitis may be recurrent and lead to dull periocular pain
   - **headaches, migraine.** Often a strong family history
   - **ophthalmic shingles.** Neuralgic pain following shingles may be severe and last for years.

EYE EXAMINATION

External

- erythema or fullness of the periocular tissues – consider periorbital or orbital cellulitis (see p. 147–149)
- palpate the temporal arteries – if tender, non-pulsatile or nodular, consider temporal arteritis (see p. 74–75)
- facial and scalp scars from trauma or previous ophthalmic shingles.

Lids

- feel the lid margins for cysts or styes – these are often less visible in dark-skinned individuals and may be acutely tender (Fig. 3.1).

Visual Acuity

- document this for each eye individually with glasses if worn, or with a pinhole (need a pinhole? see p. 2) if patient has not brought glasses.

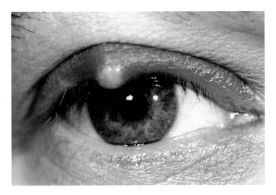

Fig. 3.1 Meibomian gland – infected lesions may be more difficult to spot in dark-skinned individuals.

Pupils

- an afferent pupil defect (see p. 7) may occur in optic neuritis or lesions compressing the optic nerve
- if pupil is dilated look for evidence of a 3rd nerve palsy* (see p. 109) which may be secondary to a cerebral aneurysm and is a **neurosurgical emergency** – headache and ptosis (drooping eyelid) may be present (Fig. 3.2)
- irregular non-reacting pupil – consider uveitis (see p. 35) where the iris is stuck to the underlying lens (Fig. 3.3) or raised intraocular pressure in acute glaucoma, particularly if the patient is in severe pain.

Eye Movements

- double vision occurs if eye movements are restricted – usually following a nerve palsy (see p. 108) or orbital mass (see p. 167).

Cornea

- stain the cornea with dilute fluorescein (make sure contact lenses are removed first) and look for foreign bodies or abrasions (see p. 27, 24) as the eye may appear normal despite these conditions in the early stages.

Fundus

- usually no fundus findings in the absence of trauma or previous surgery but hemorrhages may be visible in diabetics, hypertensives and those with ocular ischemia.

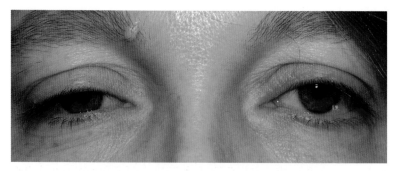

Fig. 3.2 Sudden onset ptosis – especially with a headache should be considered a 3rd nerve palsy due to an aneurysm until proved otherwise – the ptosis may initially be quite subtle.

---

*Note that the 3rd nerve palsy does not need to be 'complete' – the pupil may be uninvolved and no extraocular muscles may be involved initially.

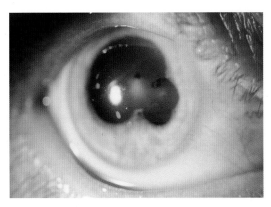

Fig. 3.3   This pupil is dilated and shows iris adhesions to the underlying lens – posterior synechiae – these are not usually apparent in the undilated pupil, which in acute iritis is miosed (constricted).

TEMPORAL ARTERITIS

Management

This is fully discussed on page 75.

SINUSITIS

Features

- often a recurrent history of sinusitis
- pain may be acute or chronic, often relapsing.

Examination

1. Ensure that visual acuity, pupils and eye movements are normal and **document findings.**
2. Tap with your index finger over the frontal and maxillary sinuses – tenderness supports the diagnosis.

Management

1. X-ray the paranasal and periorbital sinuses if the diagnosis is in doubt.
2. Start oral antibiotics such as Magnapen 500 mg four times daily orally for 10 days.

Referral and Follow Up

- **double vision or a pupil defect.** Discuss with ophthalmologist urgently

■ **no ocular findings but sinusitis suspected.** Referral not required; however patient should reattend immediately should visual symptoms develop or if symptoms of pain do not improve within 48 hours

■ frequent recurrences of sinusitis. ENT outpatients.

MIGRAINE

Features

■ may be typical with headache, nausea and visual aura, classically zig-zag lights which move progressively across the visual field (fortification spectra) – affects both eyes but patient may not notice this

■ pain is usually acute, unilateral, and may last for days

■ variants include sudden, usually transient loss of vision involving whole or part of visual field which may become permanent due to retinal or cerebral arterial spasm

■ headache may not be present

■ frequently strong family history

■ if optic disc swollen, headache and transient visual loss – consider intracranial lesion or raised intracranial pressure.

Associations

■ oral contraceptive pill, chocolate, cheese, stress.

Management

1. Check blood pressure.
2. Document visual acuity and visual field to confrontation (see p. 10).
3. Check eye movements (see p. 5) and pupils (see p. 7) – a cerebral aneurysm may present with sudden-onset headache, with or without other neurological features (see p. 108 for features of 3rd nerve palsy associated with a cerebral aneurysm).
4. If patient is over 50 check ESR and look for signs and symptoms of temporal arteritis – if suspected treat appropriately (see p. 75).
5. Advise simple analgesia and rest in a quiet dark room if no other pathology is present.
6. Antiemetics if required – Maxolon 10 mg orally or intramuscular or Stemetil 5.0 mg orally or 12.5 mg intramuscular.
7. 5HT antagonist – sumatriptan (Imigran) either by mouth 50 mg, subcutaneous injection 6 mg (using auto-injector) or intranasal spray 20 mg as soon after onset as possible. Not recommended for those with a cardiovascular history or under 18 years of age.
8. Fundus examination – usually normal. If disc is swollen urgent neurological opinion required.
9. If episodes frequent, treat prophylactically.

Referral and Follow Up

- **any visual defect.** Discuss with ophthalmologist immediately
- **history of migraines with no ocular findings.** General practitioner for prophylaxis if episodes are frequent
- **new symptoms in patient over 30.** Neurology opinion required if patient already attending GP with frequent migraines despite treatment or if symptoms occur as a new finding as this may be secondary to other intracranial pathology (reactive migraine).

Pitfall

- **occipital pain.** Consider subarachnoid hemorrhage – look for a visual field defect (see p. 10) and look at optic discs which may be swollen* (Fig. 3.4) – if you suspect a bleed, discuss with neurosurgeons immediately as a small bleed may precede a large one. See also 'Transient Loss of Vision' (see p. 105).

NEURALGIA

- usually follows ophthalmic shingles but occurs in diabetics or after local trauma
- pain may be dull or stabbing and has a chronic course.

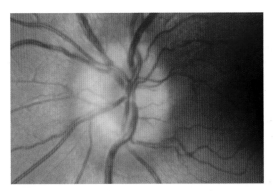

Fig. 3.4 Swollen disc in association with severe headache and visual loss may indicate subarachnoid hemorrhage – disc hemorrhage and even vitreous hemorrhage may also be present.

*A swollen disc may also be present in acute anterior ischemic optic neuropathy (Fig. 4.1), raised intracranial pressure, severe diabetic retinopathy (usually in young age group), severe hypertension, vein occlusion. Longsighted individuals (look at their glasses – act as magnifiers; (Fig. 3.5)) often have small crowded discs which look elevated, but are a normal variant.

Management

1. Consider temporal arteritis (see p. 74–75) – check ESR and CRP in a patient over 50 particularly if there are other clinical signs. (ESR may occasionally be normal in temporal arteritis. CRP – C-reactive protein.)
2. Check blood pressure and urinalysis – treat appropriately.
3. Simple analgesia – the patient frequently has not tried any simple analgesia such as paracetamol 1 g orally four times daily.
4. If history of ophthalmic shingles (see p. 43, 149–150) check for uveitis (inflammation within the eye, see p. 35) – raised intraocular pressure may be present.
5. Variable relief with
   - amitriptyline – 25 mg once daily by mouth as a starting dose (beware urinary retention, cardiotoxicity)
   - carbamazepine 100 mg at night by mouth (narrow therapeutic range and may derange full blood count)
   - transcutaneous nerve stimulation (TENS) – see 'referral' below.

Referral and Follow Up

- no follow up is required in the absence of any findings on examination
- if persistent and severe refer to neurology outpatients or pain clinic if one is available
- physiotherapist for TENS.

Discuss with or refer to physicians prior to starting amitriptyline or carbamazepine.

DIABETIC PATIENT

Pain may be acute or chronic.

1. Check blood pressure and urine.
2. Document the visual acuity with appropriate glasses if these are worn or with a pinhole (see p. 5).
3. Check eye movements and ask the patient if they see double in any position (diplopia) – diabetic neuropathy can be painful and affect the 3rd, 4th or 6th nerves (see p. 108–109).
4. Look for diabetic retinopathy (hemorrhages, exudates; Fig. 4.14) and document this – dilate pupils with tropicamide 1% one drop to each eye if required.
5. Try simple analgesia, e.g. paracetamol 1 g orally four times daily.
6. The neuralgia usually resolves spontaneously over a few days.

Referral and Follow Up

- **reduced vision, diplopia, retinopathy.** Ophthalmologist within 24 hours

- **persistent, non-resolving pain with no ocular findings.** Medical outpatients – vascular assessment may be required – usually doppler scan of carotids – (see 'ischemic pain' below)
- **new diabetics and hypertensives.** General practitioner initially.

Pitfall

- failure to recognize and refer diabetic retinopathy as untreated proliferative disease may rapidly lead to permanent visual disability.

ISCHEMIC PAIN

- usually known arteriopath
- often difficult diagnosis to make
- pain is usually chronic but may present acutely.

Management

1. Check blood pressure and urine – treat as appropriate.
2. Listen to the carotids –in the angle of the jaw for bruits and document findings – note that **no** bruit may be heard with extensive stenosis.
3. Look for retinal hemorrhages which can occur in ischemia and diabetes – particularly significant if there is marked asymmetry between each eye.
4. Start on aspirin 75 mg orally once daily unless there are contra-indications such as peptic ulceration.

Referral and Follow Up

- **all cases** – to ophthalmology outpatients where vascular assessment will be arranged if required.

SPECTACLES – INCORRECT OR ABSENT

- incorrect glasses or the need for these may lead to headache rather than localized eye pain
- patients frequently complain of 'tired eyes' particularly after prolonged reading or TV.

1. Document visual acuity with glasses if these are worn – ensure that they are wearing the correct glasses – they may be wearing their reading glasses (Fig. 3.5) for TV for example.
2. Ensure glasses are clean and not scratched.
3. If vision is reduced use a pinhole (see p. 5).
4. Improved pinhole acuity indicates the need for glasses in the majority of cases.
5. Middle-aged patients having difficulty reading may require reading glasses (presbyopia).

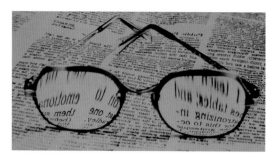

Fig. 3.5   Reading glasses often act as magnifiers – if a patient is unsure which of their spectacles to use for distance, the ones which magnify least will be correct.

Referral and Follow Up

- if vision does not improve with a pinhole refer to ophthalmology outpatient department
- all other cases – refer to optician for refraction.

Chapter 4

Visual Symptoms

This chapter refers only to conditions affecting vision.

Common Complaints

LOSS OR REDUCTION OF VISION

Ask Directly

Most patients will describe severe reduction as total loss of vision – both are included below.

ACUTE TOTAL LOSS – NO PERCEPTION OF LIGHT

■ optic nerve infarction
■ central retinal artery occlusion
■ occipital infarct
■ functional blindness – patients perceive themselves to be blind (see p. 79).

Ask Directly

■ **headache.** Jaw claudication, weight loss, scalp tenderness, shoulder girdle pain, history of polymyalgia rheumatica – all or some indicate temporal arteritis (see p. 74–75)
■ **hypertension and smoking.** Usually associated with arterial and venous occlusion

- **known arteriopath.** Angina, previous heart attack, heart valve or carotid disease – predispose to arterial occlusion (Fig. 4.2a)
- **loss of upper or lower field.** Common in non-arteritic optic neuropathy – that is, hypertension related (Fig. 1.15)
- **bilateral.** Cortical blindness if simultaneous visual loss, arterial occlusion/ischemia if one eye followed the other – often within hours or days.

OPTIC NERVE INFARCTION

Anterior Ischemic Optic Neuropathy (AION) (Fig. 4.1)

1. **Temporal arteritis (arteritic)** – blockage of the arteries supplying the optic nerve secondary to arterial inflammation.
2. **Arteriosclerotic (non-arteritic)** – blockage due to arteriolar narrowing in the elderly – particularly hypertensives, smokers and arteriopaths.

Features

- profound visual loss especially in arteritic type
- altitudinal (upper or lower) field loss common in non-arteritic group (Fig. 1.15)
- afferent pupil defect (see p. 7), swollen optic disc, hemorrhages, cotton wool spots.

Associations

- temporal arteritis – usually aged 65+
- hypertension – usually aged 45+
- arteriosclerosis, smoking, diabetes, idiopathic.

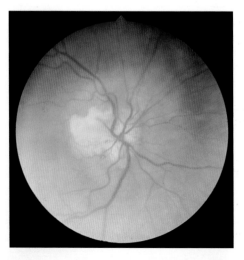

Fig. 4.1 Anterior ischemic optic neuropathy – note the pale disc and infarcted retina.

Examination and Management

1. Document visual acuity in each eye – use a pinhole if required (see p. 5).
2. Examine pupil for afferent defect and document (see p. 7).
3. Optic nerve is frequently swollen, pale and may have small hemorrhages.
4. Retina may be pale with a bright red patch at the macula if an arterial occlusion is present (see p. 76, 77).
5. Treat as temporal arteritis if suspected – features include:
   - headache
   - scalp tenderness
   - tender nodular temporal arteries
   - weight loss and malaise
   - shoulder girdle pain
   - jaw claudication – pain when eating.

INITIAL TREATMENT OF SUSPECTED TEMPORAL ARTERITIS

1. Hydrocortisone 200 mg intravenously immediately – or methyl-prednisolone 1.0–1.5 g intravenously over half an hour.
2. Oral steroid 60–80 mg if above unavailable – for 3 days and then slowly reduce.
3. Admit under ophthalmologists or physicians.
4. Take usual precautions before starting high dose steroids in hypertensives and those with a history of peptic ulceration – cover this latter group with oral ranitidine 150 mg or lansoprazole (Zoton) 30 mg twice daily.
5. Take bloods for ESR and C-reactive protein.

Management

1. Measure blood pressure and treat as required – hypertension is the most common underlying cause of AION.
2. Urine and random blood for diabetes.
3. Listen to carotids for bruits and heart sounds for murmurs – emboli arise from these sites.
4. Start aspirin 75 mg orally once daily if there are no contraindications and no evidence of temporal arteritis.
5. Advise the patient to stop smoking.

Referral and Follow Up

- temporal arteritis – admit immediately under ophthalmologist or physicians
- there is high risk of blindness in the unaffected eye without prompt adequate treatment
- all other cases – discuss immediately with ophthalmologist
- treat hypertension.

CENTRAL RETINAL ARTERY OCCLUSION (Fig. 4.2)

Features

- painless profound sudden visual loss
- afferent pupil defect
- pale retina with red macula
- embolus may be seen blocking retinal artery (Fig. 4.2a).

Associations

- arteriosclerosis – often carotid disease
- temporal arteritis
- hypertension.

Examination and Management

1. Document visual acuity.
2. Document afferent pupil defect (see p. 7).
3. Consider temporal arteritis (see p. 74, 75).
4. If retinal findings confirm diagnosis – try to re-establish arterial flow by lowering intraocular pressure (IOP) and dilating arteries:
   - intravenous Diamox 500 mg immediately – lowers IOP
   - sublingual GTN 300 μg – dilates arteries
   - massage the eye

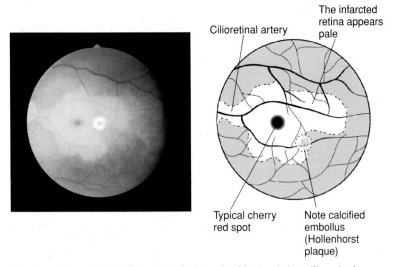

Cilioretinal artery

The infarcted retina appears pale

Typical cherry red spot

Note calcified embollus (Hollenhorst plaque)

Fig. 4.2a Central retinal artery occlusion – in this case it is a cilioretinal artery. Note the well delineated margin of the pale, infarcted retina, and the emboli seen within the arteries.

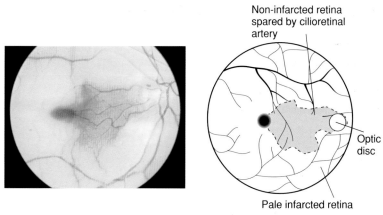

Fig. 4.2b   Central retinal artery occlusion with macular sparing.

> lie patient flat
> tell them to look towards their feet
> stand behind and with both of your index fingers 'ballot' the globe firmly through the patient's eyelids
> do this firmly – if it is not uncomfortable for the patient you are not massaging effectively
> continue for 5–10 minutes releasing intermittently.

- make patient breathe in and out from a medium-sized paper bag – raises pCO_2 and dilates arteries
- aspirin 75 mg once daily by mouth if arteriosclerotic with no evidence of temporal arteritis, and no contraindications to aspirin
- recovery is highly unlikely particularly if over two hours from onset.

Referral and Follow Up

- **to ophthalmologist in all cases**
- under 12 hours from onset – immediately refer and treat as above until transferred
- over 12 hours from onset – immediately discuss and treat as above
- features of temporal arteritis – immediately discuss and treat appropriately (see p. 74, 75) – **there is a high risk of the other eye becoming involved**
- over 12 hours old, ESR and blood pressure normal, no evidence of temporal arteritis – discuss and arrange review within 12–24 hours
- blood pressure raised, carotid bruits/heart murmurs present, no evidence of temporal arteritis – refer to physicians or vascular surgeons as appropriate for carotid doppler scan in addition to ophthalmology review within 24 hours.

Pitfall

- always consider temporal arteritis – as failure to adequately treat this condition may lead to irreversible loss of vision in the other eye within hours or days.

OCCIPITAL INFARCT (Fig. 4.3a)

Features

- sudden bilateral total or partial loss.

Associations

- hypertension
- trauma
- cerebral bleed.

Examination and Management

1. Document any visual function.
2. Pupils and fundoscopy are usually normal.
3. If field loss is not total – it is congruous – similar pattern in each eye.
4. Check blood pressure.
5. Arrange CT or MRI scan.

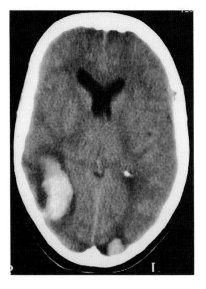

Fig. 4.3a Occipital bleed – note bilateral lesions leading to cortical blindness.

Referral and Follow Up

- discuss immediately with neurosurgeons – subdural bleed if present will need draining
- ophthalmologist once neurosurgical problem eliminated
- physicians for blood pressure control.

FUNCTIONAL LOSS

Patients complain of visual loss for which no cause can be found.

Features

- symptoms and signs which do not 'fit'
- patient often unconcerned
- 'blind' patient may still navigate around examination room with little difficulty or wince at a bright light.

Associations

- attention seeking – particularly common in adolescent girls and children with home or schooling problems
- hysteria – patient genuinely believes visual loss present, although this cannot be demonstrated
- malingering, psychiatric disturbance or associated with compensation claims.

Examination and Management

1. Document your examination findings in detail.
2. Visual acuity in each eye individually – with glasses if these are worn or pinhole if glasses have been forgotten (pinhole, see p. 2, 5).
3. Pupil reactions are normal.
4. Visual fields – may have spiral pattern (Fig. 4.3b) or be non-specific and not reproducible.
5. Shine a **bright** light into each eye without warning and observe whether they blink in the 'blind' eye.
6. Fundus – pay particular attention to the optic disc, which should be pink and healthy, and the macula (the retina temporal to the disc) which should have a flat appearance, with a small light reflex over its central part.
7. Functional loss unlikely in the elderly – consider an occipital infarct which has destroyed the visual cortex, particularly if there is a history of cardiovascular disease (Fig. 4.3a) – the pupils will be normal in an occipital infarct.
8. Ask patient to sign their name – malingerers may claim to be unable to do this, truly blind patients will retain this ability.

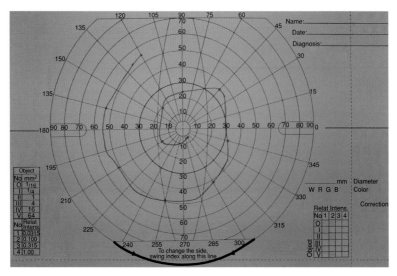

Fig. 4.3b   Spiral pattern of visual fields – typically seen in malingering.

Referral and Follow Up

- all cases – discuss with ophthalmologist immediately
- orthoptic assessment required.

Pitfalls

- functional loss is a diagnosis of exclusion, and requires detailed tests to confirm
- true pathology may appear to be functional – such as subtle macular disease in children, an occipital infarct or bilateral optic neuropathy.

ACUTE PARTIAL LOSS

central and branch retinal vein occlusion   p. 81
macular hemorrhage   p. 83
vitreous hemorrhage   p. 84
retinal detachment   p. 86
optic neuritis   p. 88
migraine   p. 68, 90

Ask Directly

- **central or overall loss.** Central loss common in macular disease – overall loss may follow vein occlusion, vitreous hemorrhage and optic neuritis

- **hypertension.** Common underlying factor in vein occlusion – malignant hypertension may lead to bilateral loss with a retinal appearance similar to diabetic retinopathy
- **history of migraine.** Visual loss may mimic a stroke – headache may not be present
- **previous age-related maculopathy.** Usually precedes a macular hemorrhage – there may be a history of central visual distortion
- **diabetic or previous vein occlusion.** Diabetic maculopathy or vitreous hemorrhage associated with new vessel formation (Fig. 4.20)
- **history of floaters and flashing lights.** Assume retinal damage – vitreous may peel off retina leading to a hemorrhage or retinal detachment (Fig. 4.8)
- **only noticed when other eye covered.** Pseudosudden loss – may have been gradual in affected eye and only noticed when good eye accidentally covered – cataract and macular lesions may present in this way with patient suggesting 'sudden' loss.

CENTRAL RETINAL VEIN OCCLUSION (CRVO); BRANCH RETINAL VEIN OCCLUSION (BRVO) (Fig. 4.4)

Features

- moderate to marked sudden, painless, usually unilateral visual loss.

Associations

- hypertension is very common – look for diabetes, raised blood viscosity (multiple myeloma, polycythemia)
- smoking
- glaucoma – chronic.

Examination and Management

1. Document visual acuity.
2. Afferent pupil defect (see p. 7) in severe cases only.
3. Fundus examination – whole retina affected in CRVO (Fig. 4.5) only part of retina affected in BRVO (Fig. 4.4).
4. Retinal hemorrhages – may be few or widespread often with cotton wool spots (patchy white retinal lesions secondary to ischemia) and blurred disc margins.
5. Raised intraocular pressure – over 21 mmHg – predisposes to vein occlusion – if you do not have experience measuring this, you are unlikely to obtain an accurate reading – leave to the ophthalmologist. If a tonopen (portable tonometer) is available – then use and document pressure.
6. Measure and treat blood pressure as required.
7. Check urine and random blood for diabetes.

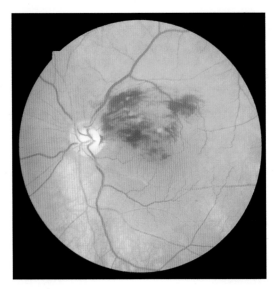

Fig. 4.4 A superotemporal branch vein occlusion – the hemorrhages and edema affect the macula region and vision is reduced. If the blockage is more peripheral vision may be spared. Note the cotton wool spots indicating ischemia.

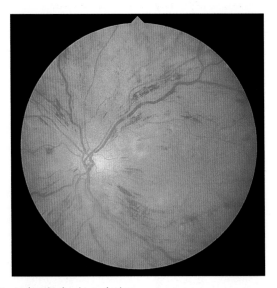

Fig. 4.5 Central retinal vein occlusion.

8. Send blood for FBC, plasma electrophoresis, blood sugar and cholesterol.
9. Advise patient to stop smoking.

Referral

- all cases – ophthalmologist within 24 hours.

MACULAR HEMORRHAGE (Fig. 4.6)

Features

- sudden or pseudosudden painless central loss with normal peripheral vision
- often preceded by central distortion of vision – typically straight lines appear wavy or have bits missing – usually in patients with age-related maculopathy
- shape is frequently circular – hence often termed 'disciform' hemorrhage (Fig. 4.6).

Associations

- age 65+ – usually spontaneous and often history of macular degeneration (see p. 98)
- younger patients – may be associated with trauma (Fig. 4.7).

Examination and Management

1. Document visual acuity – may be severely reduced.
2. Pupil reaction is normal.
3. Dilate pupil with tropicamide 1% if required.

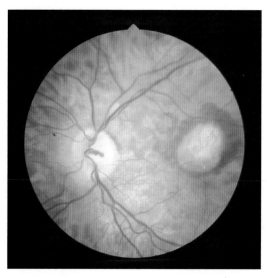

Fig. 4.6   Disciform macular hemorrhage with central scarring.

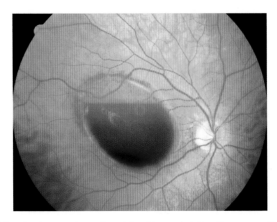

Fig. 4.7 Macular hemorrhage breaking through into vitreous cavity – typical 'boat shape' – traumatic in this case but often seen in diabetics with proliferative retinopathy.

4. Fundus examination – macular bleed, or if older, fibrosis (Fig. 4.6).
5. May be associated vitreous hemorrhage (Fig. 4.8).

Referral and Follow Up

■ **profound loss** – ophthalmologist within 48 hours – there is no useful treatment at this stage – ask about visual distortion in the other eye (see below)
■ **visual distortion or blurring** – discuss immediately with ophthalmologist – on rare occasions laser treatment can arrest progression to profound loss.

VITREOUS HEMORRHAGE (Fig. 4.8)

Features

■ moderate to profound painless visual loss usually preceded by floaters, 'cobwebs' or flashes
■ may have a history of recurrence.

Associations

■ advanced diabetic eye disease – proliferative retinopathy (see p. 100)
■ torn retinal blood vessel secondary to vitreous gel peeling away from its normal retinal attachments – posterior vitreous detachment (PVD, Fig. 4.8)
■ old retinal vein occlusion
■ trauma – direct or via any Valsalva maneuver – coughing, sneezing, lifting heavy weights.

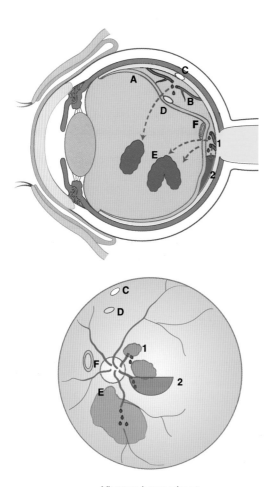

Vitreous haemorhage

2 main causes:
  PROLIFERATIVE DIABETIC RETINOPATHY
  1. New vessels at disc frequently bleed
  2. Pre-retinal haemorrage with flat upper edge - this is a pool
     of blood in front of the retina and held in place by the
     vitreous gel

POSTERIOR VITREOUS DETACHMENT
  A. Vitreous gel peels away from its internal attachment
     to the retina
  B. It may pull on and rupture a peripheral blood vessel
  C. A hole may be pulled out of the retina
  D. The segment of retina pulled out (operculum) may be
     seen floating in the vitreous
  E. Haemorhage into the vitreous occurs
  F. Ring of condensed vitreous previously attached to
     optic nerve head

Fig. 4.8 Vitreous hemorrhage.

Examination and Management

1. Document visual acuity.
2. Trauma related (see p. 112).
3. Afferent pupil defect (see p. 7) suggests underlying retinal detachment or old vein occlusion.
4. Poor visibility of the retina with loss of the red reflex common.
5. Dilate pupils with tropicamide 1%.
6. Blood may be seen floating in vitreous gel.
7. Look at retina of other eye – retinal hemorrhages may indicate diabetic retinopathy.
8. Check urine and blood sugar if patient is not a known diabetic.

Referral and Follow Up

- trauma – ophthalmologist immediately
- all others – refer within 24 hours
- known diabetics with recurrent vitreous hemorrhage — refer for early ophthalmology review – advise avoidance of strenuous activity
- new diabetics – discuss with physicians and arrange review with ophthalmologist – 24 hours.

Pitfalls

- failure to examine opposite eye for retinal pathology such as proliferative retinopathy
- the vitreous hemorrhage may mask an underlying retinal detachment or rarely a melanoma.

RETINAL DETACHMENT (Fig. 4.9)

Features

- often preceded by 'flashes' or 'cobwebs' or a shower of floaters
- painless loss of part or whole of visual field
- may progress over several days
- often described as a shutter or curtain coming down over the eye
- visual distortion rather than visual loss may occur.

Associations

- myopia or short-sightedness – look through the patient's glasses – a myopic correction makes objects look smaller (Fig. 4.10a)
- posterior vitreous detachment (detachment of the vitreous jelly from its normal retinal attachments) (Fig. 4.10b)
- blunt trauma – old or new
- previous eye surgery for detached retina or cataract.

Examination and Management

1. Document the visual acuity.

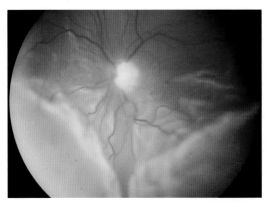

Fig. 4.9   Retinal detachment – if recent, the retina may be mobile.

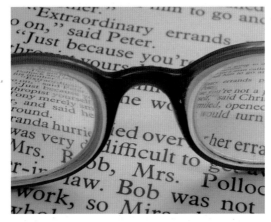

Fig. 4.10a   Myopic correction – note glasses make objects seem smaller.

2. An afferent pupil defect may be present in a large detachment.
3. Fundus examination may reveal grayish-colored mobile retina, sometimes with a rippled surface (Fig. 4.9).
4. In long-standing cases the retina may be less mobile, translucent and difficult to visualize.
5. Examine retina of other eye.

Referral and Follow Up

■ immediately discuss with ophthalmologist if symptoms are new
■ if symptoms over 3 days old – discuss and refer within 24 hours
■ fresh detachments with good visual acuity (macula still attached) require admission and surgery soon to preserve central vision.

FLASHES, FLOATERS AND COBWEBS

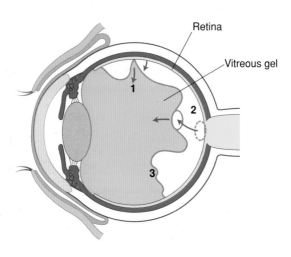

1 Vitreous detachment
Vitreous gel peels away from retina.
The mechanical traction on the retina is
seen as a flash of light (photopsia)

2 Vitreous is slightly 'thicker' at the optic disc.
If it detaches, a full or partial 'ring' may be
seen by patient

3 Folds in the vitreous gel often appear as 'cobwebs'
or 'spiders' in the patient's vision

Note: Floaters flick across the visual field
with eye movements.

A fixed defect which follows eye movements
may be a macular lesion (see p. 83,98).

Fig. 4.10b   Flashes, floaters and cobwebs.

Pitfall

■ failure to examine the other eye which may also have a detachment.

OPTIC NEURITIS (ON)

Features

■ usual age 20–40
■ vision may be normal or grossly reduced

- reduction in color perception – particularly red
- reduction in light brightness – light is brighter in normal eye
- discomfort with eye movements.

Associations

- usually none – one episode of optic neuritis with no other neurological signs **does not** indicate multiple sclerosis
- post viral – usually upper respiratory infection in children
- if previous history of neurological signs or symptoms – characteristically limb paresthesia and weakness, or previous optic neuritis, then demyelinating disease may be present.

Examination

1. Document visual acuity in each eye.
2. Gently press eye through eyelids – pain often associated with neuritis.
3. Ask patient to move eyes to extremes of gaze – often painful.
4. Check pupil for afferent defect (see p. 7) – may not be present.
5. Red saturation reduced – ask patient to compare bright red object between eyes (Fig. 2.42b) – the affected eye will often see things 'darker' (Fig. 4.11).
6. Check light brightness – a fluorescent light often appears less bright in affected eye.
7. Visual field (see p. 10) may have central and peripheral loss.
8. Ocular examination otherwise normal.
9. Optic disc may be swollen – but usually **normal**.

Management

There are three main scenarios.

1. Unilateral, other eye normal
    - no treatment
    - spontaneous resolution usual over 6 weeks.

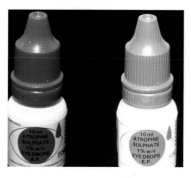

Fig. 4.11   Optic neuritis – a red object appears darker in the affected eye. Courtesy of Martindale Pharmaceuticals.

2. Severe unilateral, other eye previously affected with reduced vision
   - admit under physicians or ophthalmologists
   - pulsed intravenous methylprednisolone 1–1.5 g alternate days, three pulses total.
3. Bilateral
   - as for 2 – above.

Referral and Follow Up

- for 1. above – ophthalmologist within 24 hours
- 2. and 3. above – immediate referral to ophthalmologist or physician.

Pitfalls

- non-resolving 'optic neuritis' may indicate a space-occupying lesion
- sinusitis may be underlying cause – image if in doubt
- **do not give oral steroids alone** – if given initially these may reduce the long-term visual prognosis.

MIGRAINE

Features

- sudden usually transient loss of whole or part of visual field which may become permanent
- headache may not be present
- visual aura of migraine may occur – classically zig-zag lights which move progressively across the visual field (fortification spectra)
- vision is usually normal between episodes – profound loss may occur due to retinal arterial spasm – and even cerebral infarct
- visual field examination (see p. 10) may reveal a sector defect.

Associations

- oral contraceptive pill
- chocolate, cheese, stress
- often strong family history.

Examination and Management

1. Document visual acuity.
2. Check and document fields to confrontation (see p. 10).
3. Check blood pressure.
4. If over 50 years check ESR and consider temporal arteritis (see p. 74–75).
5. Examine for carotid bruits, heart murmurs and atrial fibrillation.
6. Fundus examination is usually normal.
7. Treat migraine if recurrent.

Referral

- if typical migraine treat as such – review if fails to resolve or worsens over 24 hours
- discuss with ophthalmologist and refer within 24 hours provided there is no evidence of temporal arteritis (see p. 75)
- if recurrent and patient over 30 – refer to neurologist – migraine presenting at this stage for the first time may be secondary to intracranial pathology.

CHRONIC LOSS

Ask Directly

- **deterioration – slow or fast**
  cataract, age-related degeneration, chronic glaucoma and nutritional amblyopia deteriorate over months and years – rarely over a few weeks
  keratoconus – initially slow with late stage acute deterioration – often with discomfort (Figs 4.12, 4.13)
  determine pattern of field loss if present (see p. 10)
- **central or peripheral loss.** Central visual loss indicates macular disease, peripheral loss glaucoma, and both together cataract – either may be present in a space-occupying lesion – particularly in cases of unexplained field loss
- **central loss preceded by distorted vision.** Typical of macula degeneration – straight lines appear wavy – e.g. door or window frames
- **increasing difficulty in sunlight or with reading.** Common in cataract, onset of presbyopia (long sight developing in 40+ age group) and old glasses
- **diabetic.** Diabetic maculopathy leads to chronic reduction in central acuity (Fig. 4.14)
- **after cataract surgery.** Thickening of the membrane supporting the lens implant can occur slowly over months or years (Fig. 4.15a–c)
- **trauma.** Past trauma may lead to future cataract and glaucoma
- **family history.** Common with glaucoma and those with early cataract – under 55 years
- **alcohol, smoking and poor diet.** A combination of these can lead to toxic or nutritional amblyopia.

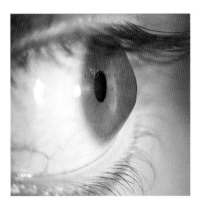

Fig. 4.12 Keratoconus – the cornea bulges into a conical shape – this process is painless but associated with slow reduction in visual acuity – and frequent change in glasses prescription.

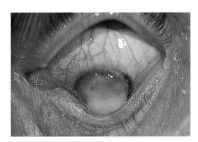

Fig. 4.13 Acute hydrops – advanced keratoconus – the distorted cornea develops 'cracks' on the inner surface and allows aqueous to suddenly penetrate the corneal stroma – painful and sudden.

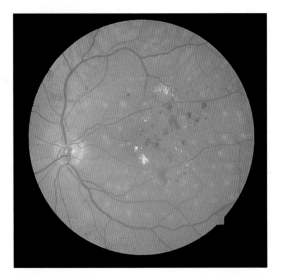

Fig. 4.14 Diabetic maculopathy leads to chronic reduction in central acuity. The pale round lesions on the left and above are recent laser burns. The white central irregular lesions are hard exudates.

Thickened posterior capsule after cataract
extraction and lens implant

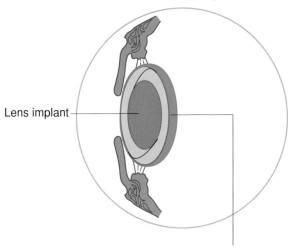

Lens implant

Posterior capsule (original membrane
surrounding cataract) thickened and opaque

a

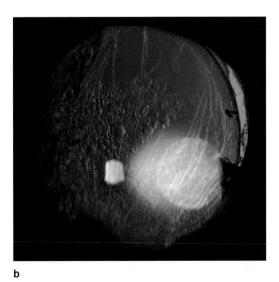

b

Fig. 4.15a,b Posterior capsule thickening after cataract surgery. Part b
reproduced with permission from Kanski J J, 2003, Clinical Ophthalmology: A
Systemic Approach, Butterworth-Heinemann.

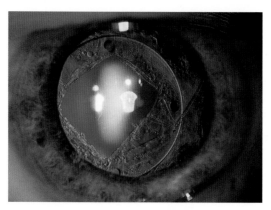

Fig. 4.15c   The membrane behind the lens implant after cataract surgery (posterior lens capsule) can thicken and lead to gradual reduction in vision – usually months to years after surgery. In this case the membrane has been opened using a YAG laser.

CATARACT (Fig. 4.16a,b)

Features

- most common cause of chronic visual loss
- most cases age related – senile cataract
- may affect distance or near vision or both – may be unilateral
- glare and shadowing around objects common.

Examination and Management

1. Document visual acuity – use appropriate glasses if worn.
2. Use pinhole (see p. 5) if patient has forgotten glasses.
3. Look at red reflex through pupils (Fig. 1.12); if obscured, may indicate cataract.
4. Fundus examination may be difficult or distorted.
5. Use slit lamp if available – lens opacity may be easily seen.
6. Dilate with tropicamide 1% if pupil is small.

Referral and Follow Up

- routine ophthalmology outpatients
- rarely, a very mature lens may leak lens protein and lead to uveitis or glaucoma – pain will then be the presenting symptom.

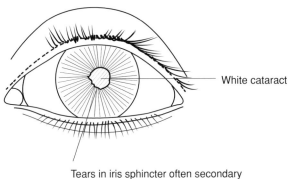

White cataract

Tears in iris sphincter often secondary
to blunt trauma

a

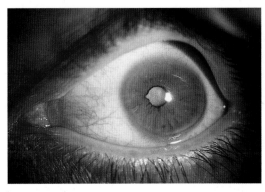

b

Fig. 4.16a,b Cataract – an advanced one may be easily seen even through a small pupil – early cataract may be very subtle. Note the irregular iris margin – these small tears are ruptures in the iris sphincter muscle secondary to blunt trauma (see p. 114) – a cause of unilateral or presenile cataract.

GLAUCOMA

Features (Fig. 4.17)

ACUTE GLAUCOMA IS PAINFUL AND DEALT WITH ON PAGE 41.

- chronic glaucoma is painless and is usually found on routine testing
- field loss is usually only noticed when central vision is affected
- family history common
- allergic reaction to drops may occur (see p. 46, 50).

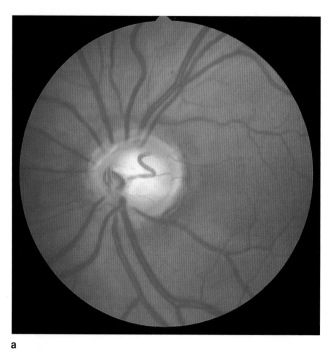

a

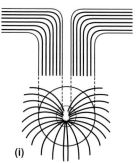

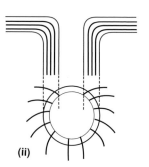

(i)

(ii)

Normal disc
"filled" with retinal nerve fibers -
little room for central cup

Glaucomatous disc
with only a few nerve fibers
spread around the edge of the
large central cup

Note: Be aware that myopic (short sighted) people may have bigger
discs and these may appear to be cupped. Conversely long
sighted people (hypermetropes) have smaller eyes and discs
and the nerve fibers may bunch up as they exit through the
small disc. This may look like disc swelling or papilledema.

b

Fig. 4.17a, Pale cupped optic disc in advanced chronic glaucoma – compare
this with a normal disc (Fig. 4.17c). **b,** Normal versus glaucomatous disc.

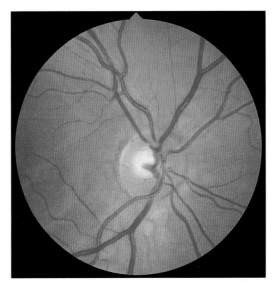

Fig. 4.17c   Normal optic disc – compare this with the cupped glaucomatous disc (Fig. 4.17a).

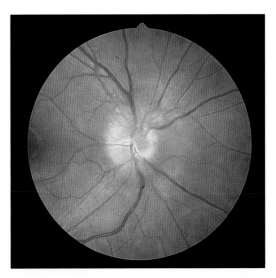

Fig. 4.17d   Swollen optic disc – in this case papillitis – papilledema looks similar and is usually bilateral.

Examination

1. Document visual acuity.
2. Test visual fields (see p. 10); if defect present then glaucoma is likely to be advanced.
3. Check intraocular pressure if tonometer available.
4. Optic disc may be pale and cupped, or just notched (Fig. 4.17).

Management, Referral and Follow Up

- discuss with ophthalmologist within 48 hours if marked field loss or disc cupping
- ensure patient is in fact using glaucoma drops if they already have these.

AGE-RELATED MACULAR DEGENERATION (Fig. 4.18)

Features

- usually over 65 years – can occur earlier
- gradual reduction in central acuity – difficulty reading and recognizing people
- sudden deterioration associated with macular hemorrhage (Fig. 4.6)
- peripheral vision usually normal.

Examination

1. Document visual acuity – use glasses if appropriate.
2. Using a pinhole may worsen visual acuity.

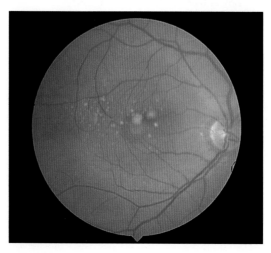

Fig. 4.18 Small submacular hemorrhage associated with visual distortion and age-related maculopathy (drusen).

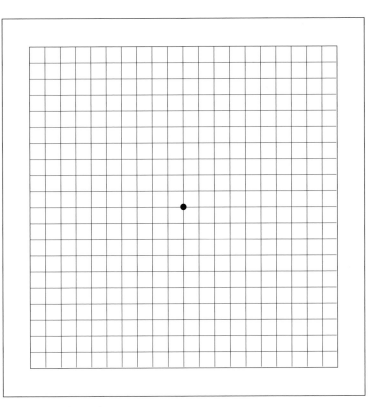

Fig. 4.19 Amsler grid
1. cover one eye and hold chart at normal reading distance
2. ask patient to look at black spot in center of grid
3. with gaze fixed on central spot – patient should be aware of grid lines being straight – missing or distorted areas indicate maculopathy.

3. Ask patient to look at a door frame – if distorted, indicates maculopathy.
4. A more sensitive test uses a grid (Fig. 4.19).
5. Pupil examination is normal – however is often miosed (small) in the elderly.
6. If the pupil is small – dilate with tropicamide 1%.
7. Look at the macula – to do this, ask the patient to look directly at the ophthalmoscope light or find the optic disc, and look temporally about two to three disc diameters.
8. Cataract may also be present in this population.

Management, Referral and Follow Up

■ if sudden reduction or distortion – discuss with ophthalmologist immediately – very rarely laser treatment can help arrest deterioration

- no acute management required in chronic cases – routine ophthalmology outpatients
- optician – low visual aid assessment – routine.

DIABETIC RETINOPATHY AND MACULOPATHY
(Figs 4.20a,b, 4.21a,b)

Features

- maculopathy leads to central visual loss
- background retinopathy is symptom free
- vitreous hemorrhage is usually associated with proliferative retinopathy.

Examination and Management

1. Document visual acuity – including reading acuity using reading glasses if required.
2. Dilate with tropicamide 1%.
3. Retinal hemorrhages and exudates are common.
4. The macula – retina temporal to the disc may have been 'thickened' with edema and have hemorrhages and exudates.
5. Ocular examination is otherwise usually normal.
6. Vitreous hemorrhage (see p. 84).

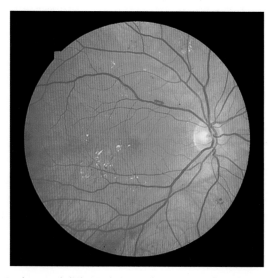

Fig. 4.20a Background diabetic retinopathy and maculopathy – note exudates spreading towards the fovea.

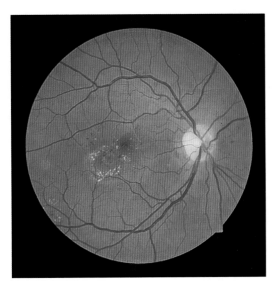

Fig. 4.20b   Focal maculopathy.

Referral and Follow Up

- vitreous hemorrhage – ophthalmologist within 24 hours
- all other cases – ophthalmologist within 48 hours.

AFTER CATARACT SURGERY

Features

- gradual reduction in clarity with haze or net curtain effect in posterior capsule thickening – this is the membrane on which the lens implant rests (see Fig. 4.15, pp 93–94)
- central loss in macular edema (Fig. 4.21).

Examination

- document visual acuity
- fundus examination difficult and distorted if membrane thickening present
- easily seen with slit lamp as semi-opaque sheet behind lens implant
- if capsule is clear – look at macula – abnormal appearance may indicate macular edema – particularly if cataract surgery has been complicated.

Management, Referral and Follow Up

- routine to ophthalmology outpatients
- posterior capsule thickening may require a YAG laser capsulotomy (see Fig. 4.15, pp 93–94)

Macula edema

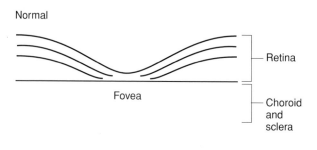

Normal

Fovea

Retina

Choroid
and
sclera

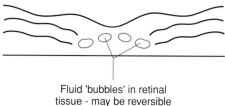

Early macula edema

Fluid 'bubbles' in retinal
tissue - may be reversible

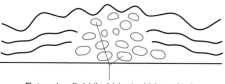

Advanced macula edema

Extensive fluid 'bubbles' within retinal
tissue - permanent reduction in
vision usual

Fig. 4.21a Macula edema.

- chronic macular edema is usually untreatable
- no follow up required.

OLD GLASSES

Features

- slow reduction in acuity or intolerant of glasses
- common in middle age when reading glasses require upgrading.

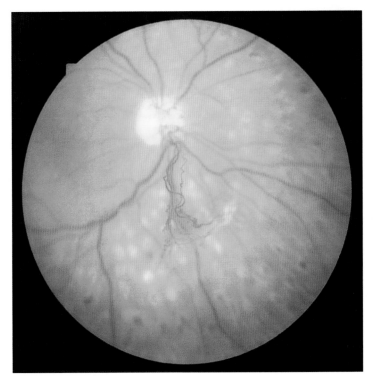

Fig. 4.21b Proliferative diabetic retinopathy – new vessels growing into vitreous from the optic disc – peripheral laser burns are also visible.

Management

1. Nil – refer to optician for refraction.
2. If child – ensure frame fits – as if uncomfortable child will reject – refer to optician.

TOXIC OR NUTRITIONAL AMBLYOPIA

Features

- gradual reduction in central acuity and color vision
- poor diet, smoker, high alcohol intake.

Examination and Management

1. Document visual acuity.
2. Document field to confrontation (see p. 10).
3. Ocular examination is otherwise usually normal.

4. Optic discs may be slightly pale.
5. Send blood for vitamin B12 and folate.

Referral and Follow Up

- ophthalmologist within 48 hours
- dietary advice and stop smoking
- course of B12 and folic acid supplements.

CENTRAL VISUAL LOSS

Dealt with Under Either Acute or Chronic Loss

SPACE-OCCUPYING LESION (SOL) OR CEREBROVASCULAR ACCIDENT (CVA)

Features

- field defect depends upon site of lesion (Fig. 1.15c,d)
- CVA defect is sudden, SOL gradual.

Examination and Management

1. Document visual acuity.
2. Document field to confrontation (see p. 10).
3. Full neurological examination – cranial nerve palsies may occur in SOL (see p. 108–110).
4. Optic disc swelling indicates papilledema and SOL until proved otherwise.
5. Optic nerve(s) may be pale or cupped.
6. Ocular examination often otherwise normal.
7. Check blood pressure and treat as required.
8. Consider migraine (see p. 68, 90) – field loss may be transient or permanent.

Referral and Follow Up

- neurosurgery within 24 hours if SOL suspected
- physicians within 24 hours for CVA.

Pitfall

- bilateral temporal field loss (the patient may complain of 'bumping into things' to the side) indicates a tumor of the optic chiasmal region until otherwise proven, particularly in the presence of optic disc pallor.

TRANSIENT LOSS OF VISION

Features

- transient loss lasting from a few seconds to minutes with recovery is usually related to retinal ischemia – common in the elderly
- visual loss may be total or partial prior to recovery – and may spread 'like a shutter coming down'
- green color prior to loss may be described by patient
- migraine may lead to transient or permanent loss from cerebral ischemia
- bilateral loss is usually related to reduction in cerebral blood flow
- pain – not usually a feature but headache may occur in carotid insufficiency, migraine and temporal arteritis.

Main Causes

1. Platelet or cholesterol emboli in the retinal circulation thrown off from atherosclerotic carotid arteries.
2. Atrial fibrillation.
3. Vertebro-basilar or gross carotid insufficiency leads to bilateral simultaneous transient loss.
4. Temporal arteritis.
5. Migraine.
6. Angle closure (acute) glaucoma.
7. Papilledema.
8. Benign intracranial hypertension – young, usually obese, female.

Examination and Management

1. Document visual acuity with glasses if worn or with pinhole (see p. 5).
2. Palpate temporal arteries – if solid, non-pulsatile or tender in patient over 50 suspect temporal arteritis (see p. 74–75).
3. Assess and document any gross field defect in each visual quadrant (see p. 10).
4. Pupils – usually normal.
5. Dilate with tropicamide 1% – avoid this however if patient describes haloes around lights with transient visual loss – or if patient is very long sighted (look at their glasses – the one they use for distance will look like a strong magnifying glass – (Fig. 3.5) – these features suggest glaucoma (see p. 41).
6. Look for retinal emboli which appear as white specks within the retinal arterioles (Fig. 4.2a) adjacent to optic disc or more peripherally.

7. Aspirin 75 mg daily if emboli present and no contraindications.
8. Listen to carotids (in the angle of the jaw) for bruits – and heart for murmurs.
9. Swelling of one or both optic discs may indicate papilledema or infarction – bilateral disc swelling is papilledema until proved otherwise – undertake full neurological examination.

Referral and Follow Up

- temporal arteritis suspected (see p. 74–75)
- papilledema – discuss with and refer immediately to the neurosurgeons
- heart murmur, carotid bruit or atrial fibrillation – discuss with the physicians for cardiovascular work up
- emboli visible on fundoscopy – treat as above and refer for carotid doppler imaging and echocardiogram
- no cause found – discuss with ophthalmologist immediately and arrange assessment within 24 hours.

FLASHES, FLOATERS AND COBWEBS (Figs 4.10b [see p. 88], 4.22)

Features

- **flashes or sparks of light (photopsia)** – response to mechanical traction on the retina – typical in:
  posterior vitreous detachment (PVD) – when the vitreous gel peels away from the retinal surface
  retinal detachment – RD – which may follow PVD as a result of a hole being pulled in the retina (Fig. 4.10b)
  migraine-related visual aura usually consists of a zig-zag line of light which flickers and moves across the visual field rather than isolated flashes
- **floaters** – opacities in the vitreous gel which sway in front of the patient's field of vision with eye movements – occur following:
  posterior vitreous detachment (PVD) – see above
  hemorrhage within the vitreous usually in diabetics, PVD or following trauma (Fig. 4.8)
  longstanding – particularly in myopes (short-sighted patients) who can see these more distinctly
- **'Cobwebs' and 'flies'** are floaters – this is a characteristic description by patients, who describe trying to wipe away a cobweb or thread which appears to hang in front of their face (Fig. 4.22).

Examination and Management

Search for gross defects only and document these if found.

1. Document visual acuity in each eye with glasses if worn or using a pin hole (see p. 5) if patient has forgotten glasses.
2. Check visual fields (see p. 10) for any gross defect which may indicate retinal detachment.

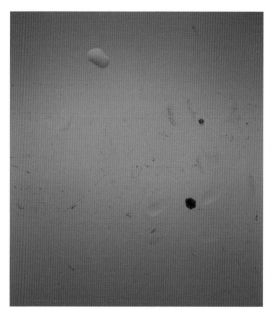

Fig. 4.22 Floaters – appear as semi-transparent circles and tubes – described as cobwebs or flies by the patient – usually noticed against a bright plain background.

3. Dilate with tropicamide 1% to each eye.
4. Look for retinal detachment (see p. 86 and Fig. 4.9) or vitreous opacities including hemorrhage (Fig. 4.8).
5. A detailed examination for peripheral retinal damage can only be undertaken by an ophthalmologist.

Referral and Follow Up

- if retinal detachment or vitreous hemorrhage seen – discuss immediately with ophthalmologist
- all other cases that are not typically migraine related – usually a long history of similar symptoms – should be referred to the ophthalmologist within 24 hours.

DOUBLE VISION – DIPLOPIA

Main Causes

1. Ischemia
   - age
   - hypertension
   - diabetes.
2. Trauma

3. Compressive
- thyroid eye disease (see p. 53)
- aneurysm usually affecting the 3rd or 6th cranial nerve
- mass lesion.

Ask Directly

- painful or painless
  painful sudden onset 3rd nerve palsy may be due to an intracranial aneurysm
  immediately discuss with neurosurgeons
- hypertensive, diabetic or known arteriopath
  all commonly associated with ischemia
  can affect 3rd, 4th or 6th nerves leading to diplopia
  may be painful or painless
- is double vision horizontal, vertical or a mixture of both (see p. 5, 'Eye movements')
- horizontal diplopia – images side to side
  usually 6th nerve palsy
  occasionally breakdown of longstanding squint
  cerebral infarct or mass
- vertical diplopia – images above each other or skewed
  4th nerve palsy – traumatic, ischemic or breakdown of congenital weakness
  3rd nerve palsy – ischemic or secondary to aneurysm
  thyroid eye disease (see p. 53)
  mass behind eye
  blow-out fracture (see p. 123)
- thyroid problems (see p. 53)
  thyroid eye disease may have a gradual or sudden onset
  symptoms may include tremor, heat intolerance, weight loss, poor temper, palpitations
  diplopia from mechanical restriction of extraocular muscles
  most common in middle-aged women
- trauma (see p. 114)
  blunt injury to orbit may lead to blow-out fracture as above
  orbital hematoma may restrict globe movement
  surgical trauma – particularly after retinal detachment repair
- paresthesia elsewhere or history of optic neuritis (see p. 88)
  in younger patients consider demyelinating disease
- ptosis – intermittent or prolonged drooping of upper lid
  consider myasthenia gravis – this is rare
  if sudden – consider 3rd nerve palsy – even if pupil is normal (see p. 110)
- does diplopia or shadowing persist even if one eye is covered
  monocular diplopia – may indicate cataract.

Examination

1. Trauma (see p. 112).
2. Document visual acuity in each eye with appropriate glasses or pinhole.
3. Ask patient to look straight ahead and document:
   - whether the eyes are both looking straight ahead
   - type of double vision – horizontal or vertical or a mix of these
4. Eye movements
   - limited lateral gaze or increasing horizontal diplopia when asked to look to the side usually indicates 6th nerve palsy
   - eye fixed in 'down and out' position indicates 3rd nerve palsy – usually in association with a ptosis on the same side.
5. Eyelids – if unilateral ptosis - suspect 3rd nerve palsy
   - **a painful 3rd nerve palsy indicates a cerebral aneurysm until proved otherwise – this is a neurosurgical emergency** (see p. 110).
6. Pupil
   - enlarged – suspect 3rd nerve palsy secondary to cerebral aneurysm
   - normal – diabetic or ischemic microvascular disease
   - **a normal pupil with a 3rd nerve palsy does not rule out a cerebral aneurysm.**
7. Prominent or staring eyes – may be white or injected – consider
   - thyroid eye disease – ask about systemic symptoms and family history (see p. 53)
   - orbital mass lesion (see p. 167).
8. Corneal sensation – loss or reduced sensation may be the first indication of an acoustic neuroma – particularly in association with an ipsilateral 6th nerve palsy and hearing defect.

To Check Corneal Sensation

1. Roll a small fragment of tissue to a soft point.
2. Approaching from the side so that the patient does not see the tissue approaching – touch the cornea gently – the patient should blink.
3. Compare sensation in both eyes.

Retina

- usually normal but diabetic patients may have retinopathy and swollen optic discs indicate papilledema until proved otherwise.

General Examination

- look for other injuries if trauma related
- blood pressure
- urinalysis or blood glucose for diabetes.

Management and Referral

Painful 3rd Nerve Palsy with Pupil Involvement
- transfer the patient immediately by ambulance – not by car – to neurosurgical team
- patients may die en route from aneurysmal rupture.

3rd Nerve Palsy with Normal Pupil
- admit the patient under the neurosurgeons for observation as pupil involvement may subsequently occur
- 'pupil sparing' – a normal pupil in the presence of a third nerve palsy may occur in the presence of an aneurysm. The neurosurgeons will refer to the ophthalmologists if required.

6th or 4th Nerve Palsy
- **patients under 50 years of age should be seen within 24 hours and investigated by ophthalmologist or physicians**
- if diabetic, hypertensive or known arteriopath and no other neurological signs present – arrange follow up in 5–7 days after discussing with the ophthalmologist
- reduced corneal sensation or hearing – refer to neurosurgeons within 24 hours
- discuss with physicians if newly diagnosed diabetic or hypertensive
- patient to reattend immediately if any new features develop
- temporal arteritis – may rarely present as a 6th nerve palsy (see p. 74–75).

Trau matic
- discuss immediately with ophthalmologist
- X-ray orbits and paranasal sinuses – look for a blow-out fracture – opacity in the maxillary sinus (Fig. 5.12), air in the orbit or blood in the sinuses
- treat prophylactically with systemic broad spectrum antibiotics such as oral Magnapen 500 mg four times daily in adults – if there is evidence of a blow-out fracture or an open wound is present
- check tetanus status and treat if required
- see Chapter 5 for further details on trauma management.

Children
- all children should be urgently seen by an ophthalmologist with the exception of a painful 3rd nerve palsy which must be transferred urgently to the neurosurgeons as above.

Association with Previous Neurological Deficits
- suggests demyelinating disease and should be referred to the neurologists within 48 hours.

Thyroid Eye Disease and Proptosis

- if associated with pain, reduced vision or an afferent pupil defect (see p. 7), discuss with ophthalmologist immediately
- other cases – ophthalmologist within 24 hours.

Other Cases

- cataract – monocular diplopia – the patient sees double out of one eye
- myasthenia gravis – often worse at the end of the day
- breakdown of longstanding ocular imbalance or previous surgery, e.g. after retinal detachment repair.

All of the above should have an early ophthalmology outpatient appointment arranged.

Pitfall

- failure to treat a 3rd nerve palsy with or without pupil involvement as a neurosurgical emergency.

Chapter 5

Trauma

Chemical injury – wash out eye now (see p. 112).

Note that the descriptions of penetrating and perforating are used interchangeably in this text – strictly, perforating injuries are full thickness, penetrating may be partial thickness.

CHEMICAL INJURY

Start washing out now before reading further.

Features

- alkali injuries – ammonia, cement, caustic soda and bleach can rapidly destroy the eye – alkali penetrates tissues rapidly
- acid injuries – acid penetrates less effectively than alkali and intraocular destruction is less marked.

Management

1. **Wash out immediately** (Fig. 5.1a) – before further history or examination.
2. Instill topical anesthetic such as proxymetacaine 0.5% benoxinate 0.4% or amethocaine 1.0% – this will allow more comfortable access for further examination and treatment.
3. Place patient on couch and irrigate the eyes with copious quantities of water or saline or just use a tap – just do not waste any time.
4. At least 1 liter per eye should be used – more for alkaline injuries – a 1 liter bag of saline with a drip set on maximum flow provides good irrigation. Ensure that no solid chemical particles are left in the folds of conjunctiva between the lower eyelid and the globe and underneath the

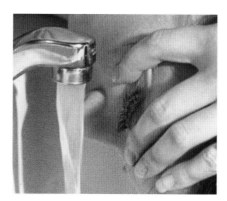

Fig. 5.1a Immediate wash out under a tap is effective – do not waste any time.

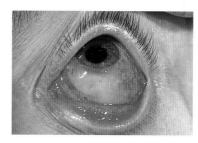

Fig. 5.1b Well-circumscribed chemical burn to cornea.

upper eyelid. Check the pH with litmus paper and stop irrigating only when neutral. **Discuss with ophthalmologist whilst washing out – continue below in mild cases.**

5. If mild irritant involved such as soaps or hairspray examine cornea after irrigation, stain with dilute fluorescein, observe under a blue light – treat as an abrasion if any staining (see p. 24).
6. Instill a drop of cyclopentolate 1% and chloramphenicol ointment 1% into affected eye(s).
7. Patch the worst eye for 24 hours.
8. Chloramphenicol ointment 1% to affected eye(s) for 5 days.

Referral and Follow Up

- acid and alkali injuries – immediate discussion with and referral to ophthalmologist
- mild chemical irritant injuries require no referral.

Pitfalls

- **failure to immediately irrigate** – do not wait to get in touch with the ophthalmologist
- inadequate irrigation – use liters and continue until neutral

- failure to remove solid debris – particularly concrete – from under the upper lid and lower conjunctival fornix.

BLUNT INJURY (Figs 5.2–5.4)

suspected globe rupture or perforating injury	p. 120
orbital hematoma – with and without view of eye	p. 121–122
double vision (suspected blow-out fracture)	p. 123
hyphema – blood level seen inside eye	p. 123

Ask Directly

- **how and when – document an accurate history.** This is particularly important in trauma – document the time of injury and the exact cause.

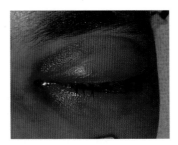

Fig. 5.2 Orbital hematoma with no view of eye.

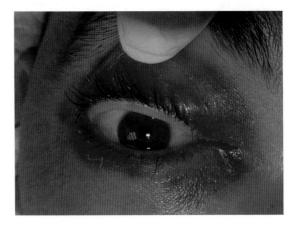

Fig. 5.3 Hematoma with view of normal-looking globe – note no pressure is exerted on the eye – the lid is retracted from the bony orbital rim.

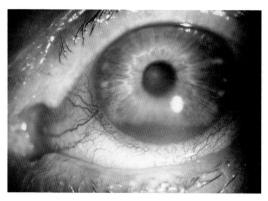

Fig. 5.4 Moderate hyphema – iris and pupil are easily visible.

Squash ball and shuttlecock injuries can be particularly severe, as they 'fit' neatly into the eye socket (Fig. 5.5). Children frequently do not tell the truth if by doing so they fear punishment. The child shown in Figs 5.6–5.9 was playing underneath a bed with a sibling and apparently knocked into a clothes pole – a benign sounding history for a life-threatening injury

■ **were they knocked out.** You will need to treat as a head injury case in addition to ocular injury

■ **is vision reduced.** This may be secondary to a corneal abrasion or internal ocular bleeding. A hyphema is a blood level seen in the front of

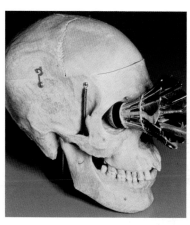
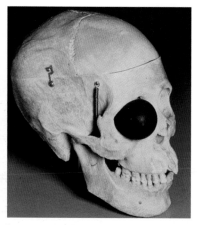

a   b

Fig. 5.5 Shuttlecocks and squash balls fit neatly inside the orbital rim – hence potential for severe injury to the globe – larger objects such as footballs hit the orbital rim first.

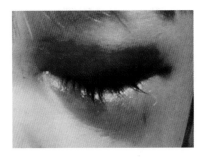

Fig. 5.6 Orbital hematoma after striking eye on end of clothes pole spike. Vision good at 6/9 (see p. 115).

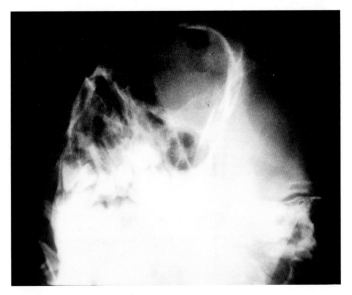

Fig. 5.7 X-ray shows gas in superior orbit.

the eye obscuring the lower portion of the iris (Fig. 5.4) it may be sufficiently severe to obscure the iris. Retinal bruising and retinal detachment may occur (Fig. 4.9)

■ **do they see double.** Orbital contents may be forced through the thin lower orbital floor into the maxillary sinus – a 'blow-out' fracture – resulting in restricted upgaze and vertical diplopia – one image vertically above the other (Fig. 5.12a).

Examination

Ensure there are no other severe non-ocular injuries that require urgent management.

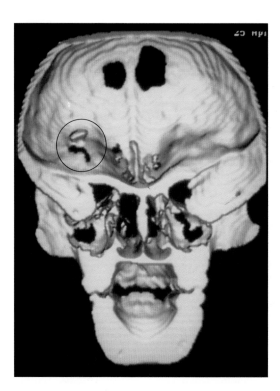

Fig. 5.8 CT scan shows hole in orbital roof – see circle.

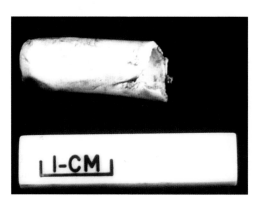

Fig. 5.9 Plastic cover from clothes pole found embedded in frontal lobe. The blunt metal tip had pierced the orbital roof underneath the upper lid and entered the frontal lobe, leaving behind this plastic sheath.

The case shown in Figs 5.6–5.9 illustrates the importance of a good history. Normal visual acuity does not rule out severe underlying trauma.

External
1. Periorbital bruising may be so severe that the eye cannot be opened. DO NOT TRY TO FORCE OPEN.
2. Feel the orbital rim for tenderness or bony fractures (Fig. 2.11d).

3. Carefully examine wounds on the lids or upper cheek – these may be sufficiently deep to involve the globe.
4. Crepitus indicates a fracture of the medial wall of the orbit.

External Globe
1. If the eye looks distorted, or it is difficult to recognize normal features it may be ruptured – **Do not attempt any further examination** – refer to ophthalmologist (Fig. 2.8).
2. Subconjunctival hemorrhage – a solid red discoloration of the normal 'white' of the eye is common and may mask an underlying globe rupture (Fig. 2.47) in severe injury.

Visual Acuity
1. Essential to document this in **each** eye individually – use a pinhole if the patient usually wears glasses.
2. Reduced vision is commonly associated with corneal abrasions (see p. 24) or hyphema (see p. 123).

Eye Movements
1. Frequently restricted as a result of orbital edema with associated double vision.

Cornea
1. Stain with fluorescein – look for an abrasion (see p. 24).
2. Full thickness corneal lacerations may occur in sharp or blunt trauma (Figs 5.10a,b, 5.11).

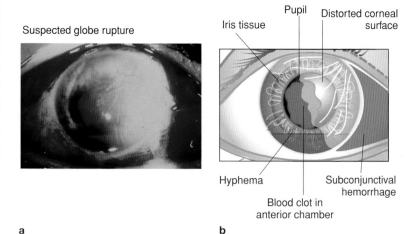

a

b

Fig. 5.10   Note marked subconjunctival hemorrhage and hyphema – the cornea looks distorted superiorly and a corneal laceration is just visible.

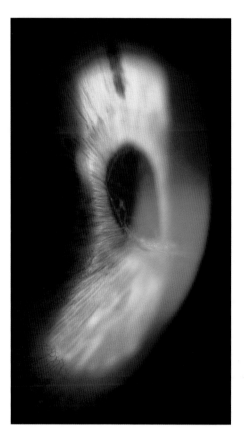

Fig. 5.11 The pupil is distorted and has prolapsed forward to the back of the cornea at the site of a perforating corneal laceration.

Iris and Pupil

1. Hyphema (Fig. 5.4) may obscure the lower part of the iris and indicates significant ocular injury.
2. Pupil distortion may be associated with perforating injury (Fig. 5.11).
3. Pupil may be dilated and sluggish as a result of trauma (traumatic mydriasis).
4. With a tight periorbital hematoma, an afferent pupil defect indicates optic nerve compression which requires urgent decompression (Fig. 5.2).

Lens

1. An opaque lens or cataract is associated with penetrating injury.
2. Severe injury may dislocate the lens.

Fundus

1. Acutely bruised retina may appear pale with scattered hemorrhages – commotio retinae.

2. Retinal detachment appears as a gray floating 'curtain' on fundoscopy (Fig. 4.9) – this may not be visible immediately following injury but can be a late consequence.

Management

All severe blunt ocular injuries must be reviewed by an ophthalmologist.

1. Immediately
   - globe rupture or suspected perforation
   - pupil defect with a dense periorbital hematoma
   - hyphema or visual loss in a child.
2. Within 24 hours – discuss immediately
   - reduced visual acuity
   - hyphema in an adult
   - lid lacerations
   - retinal hemorrhages
   - blow-out fracture
   - children with no hyphema and no visual loss.
3. Within 48 hours
   - normal eye with periorbital bruising.
4. No review required
   - minor trauma involving periorbita only with no eye involvement.

SUSPECTED GLOBE RUPTURE OR PENETRATING INJURY

Examination and Management

1. **Do not put any pressure on the globe at all or you may cause expulsion of intraocular contents.**
2. Cover eye with eye shield.
3. Document visual acuity in both eyes if injuries allow – record the fact that you have attempted to document vision even if unsuccessful – in the affected eye it may be no perception of light (NPL).
4. Do not instill any drops.
5. Cover with systemic antibiotics, e.g. intravenous cefuroxime 1 g stat.
6. Check tetanus status and treat appropriately.
7. X-ray orbit and paranasal sinuses – look for fluid levels, air or prolapsed tissue (opacity) – usually in the maxillary sinus (Fig. 5.12).
8. Keep patient fasted until seen by ophthalmologist to ensure surgery is not delayed.

Referral

- ophthalmologist immediately.

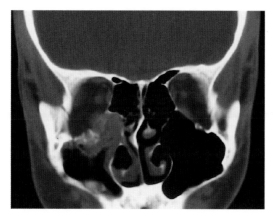

Fig. 5.12a Blow-out fracture – note prolapsed orbital contents and hemorrhage in maxillary sinus.

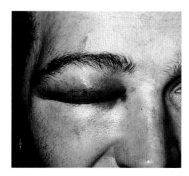

Fig. 5.12b Tight orbital tissues with hematoma – note swollen upper lid tissue.

ORBITAL HEMATOMA WITH NO VIEW OF EYE (Fig. 5.2)

Examination and Management

1. Gently place an ice pack over the orbit – AVOIDING pressure on eye – to try and reduce swelling.
2. If associated with an open skin wound check tetanus status and treat appropriately.
3. X-ray the orbit and paranasal sinuses, and look for fluid levels, air or prolapsed tissue.

Referral

- ophthalmologist immediately – assume globe rupture.

ORBITAL HEMATOMA WITH A VIEW OF THE EYE (Fig. 5.3)

Examination and Management

1. Document visual acuity.
2. Attempt to identify whether the globe is intact – the cornea should be visible as should the pupil unless there is an associated hyphema.
3. A soft distorted globe indicates a scleral rupture.
4. Check pupil for an afferent defect (see p. 7) – if present with a tight hematoma – consider optic nerve compression – if a delay is anticipated before the patient is seen by the ophthalmologist then a lateral canthotomy may prevent permanent visual loss.

Lateral Canthotomy – Procedure

1. Local anesthetic is not required – it may further increase tissue volume and pressure.
2. Clamp up to 1 cm of the outer canthus (junction between the upper and lower lids) with a pair of artery forceps for 30 seconds.
3. Cut along the line of crushed tissue with scissors.
4. Look for a hyphema and treat appropriately (see p. 123).
5. Attempt to visualize fundus even if only optic disc is seen and document this.
6. Stain cornea with fluorescein and treat any associated corneal abrasion (see p. 24).
7. If there is an open skin wound check tetanus status and treat appropriately.
8. X-ray orbit and paranasal sinuses, and look for sinus opacities.
9. Document infraorbital nerve paresthesia – numbness over upper cheek or double vision in any direction of gaze – these indicate a blow-out fracture (see p. 123).
10. Place an ice pack on the hematoma unless there is evidence of globe rupture or penetration.

Referral

- **suspected globe rupture.** Ophthalmologist immediately
- **afferent pupil defect.** Immediately to ophthalmologist especially if associated with a tight hematoma – this indicates compression of the optic nerve – see management above
- **globe intact and normal visual acuity.** Ophthalmologist within 24 hours.

Note that a sluggish or dilated pupil may be due simply to the trauma – traumatic mydriasis – however this diagnosis can only be made by the ophthalmologist.

ORBITAL BRUISING AND DOUBLE VISION – SUSPECTED 'BLOW-OUT' FRACTURE (Figs 5.12, 5.13)

Features

- double vision in upgaze and numbness of the cheek, upper lip and upper teeth indicate a 'blow-out' fracture, where orbital contents are forced through the orbital floor into the maxillary sinus.

Examination and Management

1. Treat as for 'orbital hematoma with a view of the eye' as above.
2. Cover with systemic antibiotics such as Magnapen 500 mg orally four times daily.

Referral

- ophthalmologist within 24 hours.

SUBCONJUNCTIVAL HEMORRHAGE (see p. 57 and Fig. 2.47)

Management and Referral

1. Full basic examination.
2. If globe looks intact with normal visual acuity, refer to ophthalmologist within 24 hours.
3. If vision is severely reduced, refer immediately as a subconjunctival hemorrhage may mask a globe rupture.

HYPHEMA (Fig. 5.4, p. 115)

Usually seen as a blood level in the anterior chamber (behind the cornea) as in Fig. 5.4, but may fill the eye (total hyphema).

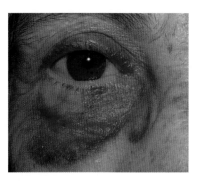

Fig. 5.13 Resolving periorbital hemorrhage – persisting double vision after swelling has subsided indicates a blow-out fracture.

Examination and Management

1. Document visual acuity.
2. Stain the cornea with fluorescein – look for an abrasion and if present treat appropriately (see p. 24).
3. Assess if globe is intact – a soft or distorted globe indicates rupture.
4. Strict bed rest reduces the risk of a rebleed which is most likely to occur 3–5 days following injury – a rebleed is usually more severe than the initial bleed and can lead to loss of the eye.
5. Predsol 0.5% three times daily and cyclopentolate 1% twice daily for secondary traumatic uveitis – only use in severe cases (more than 30% hyphema) with likelihood of more than 24 hour delay before ophthalmology review.

Referral

■ **children.** Admit under the ophthalmologists
■ **hyphema greater than one third corneal diameter.** Admit under ophthalmologists
■ **small hyphema.** If the patient is a sensible adult advise strict bed rest and arrange ophthalmological review within 24 hours; if in doubt – admit for bed rest and discuss with the ophthalmologist.

Pitfall

■ failure to advise patient of absolute necessity for bed rest **and to document this** as a rebleed can lead to loss of the eye.

LID LACERATIONS (Figs 5.14, 5.15)

1. Check for other injuries and treat appropriately – both ocular and non-ocular.
2. Assess wound depth – if full thickness the globe may also be involved.
3. If partial thickness and not through the lid margin, clean and repair with 6/0 silk, vicryl or prolene to the skin.
4. If full thickness or involving lid margin or lacrimal puncta (approximately the medial fifth of lids) leave any repair to the ophthalmologist.
5. Check tetanus status and treat appropriately.
6. Place loose, sterile dry dressing over wound.

Referral

■ any suspicion of an underlying ocular rupture or penetration (Fig. 5.17) refer immediately to ophthalmologist
■ lid lacerations can otherwise be left for 24 hours before being seen by the ophthalmologist

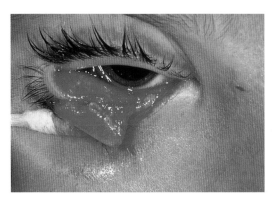

Fig. 5.14 Full thickness lid laceration.

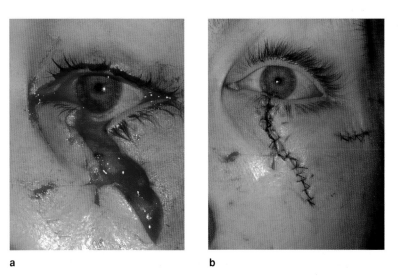

a   b

Fig. 5.15 Full thickness lid laceration, pre- (a) and postoperatively
(b) – caused by a thrown glass.

- minor lacerations with no associated ocular injury can be repaired without
  any ophthalmological referral – remove sutures after 6–10 days.

SHARP AND PENETRATING INJURIES (Figs 5.11, 5.17a)

Usual Causes

- **high-velocity particles.** Metallic fragments from 'metal on metal'
  impact such as hammering on a nail or chisel (see p. 129)

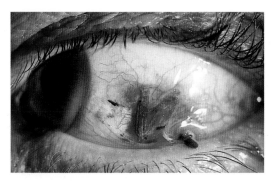

Fig. 5.16 Conjunctival laceration and wooden fragments from a tree branch – be aware of underlying scleral rupture.

Sharp and penetrating injuries

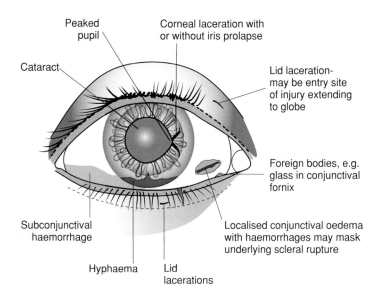

Peaked pupil

Corneal laceration with or without iris prolapse

Cataract

Lid laceration- may be entry site of injury extending to globe

Foreign bodies, e.g. glass in conjunctival fornix

Subconjunctival haemorrhage

Localised conjunctival oedema with haemorrhages may mask underlying scleral rupture

Hyphaema   Lid lacerations

Usual causes:
High-velocity particles - usually metallic fragments from metal-on-metal impact, e.g. hammering on a nail or chisel, airgun injuries.
Sharp and penetrating injuries

Fig. 5.17a Sharp and penetrating injuries.

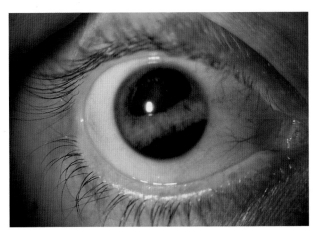

Fig. 5.17b Distorted pupil – the iris has been torn from its root inferiorly following severe blunt trauma. This is an old injury – the eye is white and quiet. Reproduced with permission from Kanski J J, 2003, Clinical Ophthalmology: A Systemic Approach, Butterworth–Heinemann.

- **glass injuries.** Assault with a broken bottle or glass, or road traffic accident (see p. 129)
- **thrown objects.** Usually children with screwdrivers, scissors and knives (see p. 129)
- **gardening.** Bending down onto a spike of a shrub or supporting stick (see p. 129).

Ask Directly

- **what activity were they doing**
- **how did it happen**
- **what time**
- **were they wearing protective goggles** – particularly important in work-related injuries.

Document answers to these questions carefully.

- **did they feel an impact and if so, where.** Look carefully for a site of entry which may be extremely small – high-velocity particles may travel through a considerable amount of tissue and still have sufficient energy to penetrate the eye (Fig. 2.11c)
- **is vision affected.** Cataract and vitreous hemorrhage may be present – **however be cautious as vision may be normal despite the presence of an intraocular foreign body.**

Examination

External

1. Blood may obscure detailed examination particularly in glass injuries associated with multiple lacerations.
2. **Carefully** attempt to clean the area and remove fragments of glass or other debris which are visible – **do not** 'dig and search' near the eye or surrounding tissue as you may cause even more injury.

Lids

1. Even small lid lacerations may be full thickness and involve the eye.
2. Look for small puncture wounds in the upper or lower lids and just below the eyebrow (Fig. 5.17a).

Visual Acuity

1. Attempt to assess and document visual acuity – but **do not put pressure on lids** to try and open them as this may prolapse intraocular tissue.
2. Vision may be reduced from intraocular hemorrhage.

Conjunctiva

1. A subconjunctival hemorrhage can mask the site of a penetrating injury.

Cornea

1. Look for blood behind the cornea – hyphema – this indicates a significant injury to the globe (Fig. 5.4).
2. The cornea may be lacerated, and iris may have prolapsed out leading to an irregularly shaped pupil (Fig. 5.11).

Pupil

1. Pupil distortion is associated with penetrating injuries affecting the front of the eye (Figs 5.11, 5.17b).
2. The pupil may be normal with posterior penetrating injuries.

Lens

1. This may become opaque shortly – usually over an hour – after being punctured.
2. Look at the red reflex (Fig. 1.12) – this may show corneal irregularities such as a laceration as well as lens and vitreous opacities.

Fundus

1. Attempt to obtain view of the retina – vitreous hemorrhage may prevent this.

X-ray

1. Orbit and paranasal sinuses as even glass fragments are occasionally radio-opaque.

2. Medicolegal difficulties may arise at a later date if this investigation is omitted.

INJURIES FOLLOWING THROWN PROJECTILES, GLASS INJURIES AND GARDENING

■ these are usually obvious – if you are in doubt as to whether penetration has occurred, treat it as a penetrating injury.

Management

1. Document visual acuity if possible.
2. If you suspect globe rupture cover with an eye shield – do not touch the eye at all and do not instill any drops.
3. If the eye appears intact carefully examine for corneal abrasions (see p. 24).
4. Examine the folds of conjunctiva in the gutter between the eye and the lower lid by making the patient look up and gently pulling the lower lid down.
5. If foreign body fragments are found here gently remove with a cotton bud – if adherent and not easily removed leave for ophthalmologist.
6. Do not evert the upper lid (see p. 32) if there is any possibility of a penetrating injury as you may expulse intraocular contents.
7. Cover with systemic or intravenous antibiotics such as cefuroxime 1 g stat intravenously or Magnapen 500 mg by mouth.
8. Check tetanus status – treat as appropriate.
9. X-ray the orbit and paranasal sinuses – a normal X-ray does not exclude an intraocular foreign body.
10. Keep patient fasted if there is a likelihood that surgery is required.

Referral

■ immediately to ophthalmologist.

Pitfalls

■ see under 'hammering, chiseling or similar' below.

HAMMERING, CHISELING OR SIMILAR

■ small, high-velocity metal fragments can penetrate the globe with little to find on examination and few, if any, symptoms
■ irreversible visual loss may only occur months later from retinal toxicity, if a ferrous intraocular foreign body is not detected early and removed.

Management

Ensure you document accident details accurately.

1. Measure and document visual acuity in each eye – remember to use a pinhole (see p. 5) if required.
2. Remove superficial corneal foreign bodies – if deep, do not attempt to remove.
3. Treat any associated corneal abrasion (see p. 24).
4. Check tetanus status and treat if appropriate.
5. X-ray the orbit.
6. Advise future use of safety goggles (Fig. 5.18).

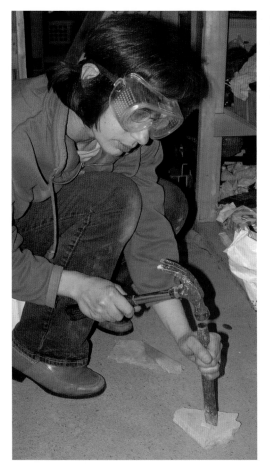

Fig. 5.18 Safety goggles can be placed over glasses and should always be worn when hammering or chiseling. Particularly in the case of metal on metal.

Referral

- **all cases must be seen by the ophthalmologist if there is any doubt about the presence of an intraocular foreign body** – a cataract may develop quite rapidly following a penetrating injury making subsequent fundus examination impossible by normal methods
- **obvious penetration** – refer immediately
- **children** – refer immediately.

Pitfalls

- an intraocular foreign body may be missed for months as the patient may be asymptomatic with initially normal vision
- the patient may re-present with an acutely inflamed eye or gradual loss of vision
- a negative X-ray – even a negative CT scan – does not rule out the possibility of an intraocular foreign body
- an MRI scan should **not** be carried out if metallic foreign bodies are suspected.

The majority of potential problems may be avoided by:

1. Accurately documenting the history.
2. Accurately documenting that a thorough examination has been undertaken.
3. Taking an X-ray of the orbit.
4. Referring to the ophthalmologist if there is any doubt.

Chapter 6

Watering Eye

ACUTE

Usually a normal physiological response to ocular irritation from any cause. If associated with:

red eye   p. 13
trauma   p. 112

CHRONIC

Features

- most cases are bilateral
- symptoms vary from intermittent nuisance to marked debility
- if associated with gritty irritable eyes – may be secondary to dry eyes or blepharitis.

Main Causes (Fig. 6.1)

Adult

1. Senile ectropion of lower lid (Figs 6.2, 8.8).
2. Stenosis (narrowing) of lacrimal punctum.
3. Blepharitis – chronic lid margin irritation (see p. 143).
4. Blockage of nasolacrimal system – usually unilateral (Fig. 6.3b).
5. Dry eye – watering may occur from irritation due to dry spots on cornea.

Child

1. Failure of canalization of nasolacrimal duct – usually under 18 months of age.
2. Congenital glaucoma – extremely rare – the eyes may look larger than normal – described mistakenly as 'beautiful big eyes'.

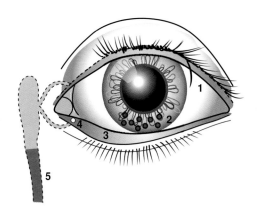

Fig. 6.1 Common causes of watering eye.

1 Foreign body or abrading eyelash.
2 Dry eye - corneal staining and irritation leads to secondary watering.
3 Ectropion
4 Stenosis of lacrimal punctum - often associated with ectropion.
5 Nasolacrimal duct blockage.

Examination

1. The bottom lid margin may not be closely applied to the eye – ectropion (Fig. 6.2), tears fill and overflow from the gutter between the eye and the poorly applied lid – common in the elderly and may occur after lower lid trauma in all age groups.
2. The medial part of the lower lid may be slightly turned out – medial ectropion – leading to drying and closure of the lacrimal puntum – the small duct responsible for tear drainage.
3. Feel for a palpable mass in the angle between the eye and nose – a mucocele (Fig. 6.4) – pressure may result in mucopus being expressed into the tear film.
4. Crusting of the lashes and erythema of the lid margin indicates blepharitis (see p. 143).
5. Stain the cornea with fluorescein and examine under a blue light on the slit lamp – fine diffuse staining may indicate a dry eye and this is associated with secondary watering. This occurs as if the tear film does not efficiently cover the whole of the cornea, dry patches may develop and the subsequent irritation leads to tear spillover.

MANAGEMENT AND REFERRAL – ADULT

Ectropion (see p. 150)
Stenosis of lacrimal punctum – as for ectropion

Ectropion

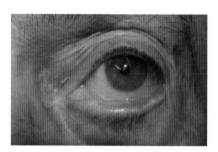

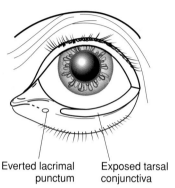

Everted lacrimal　Exposed tarsal
punctum　conjunctiva

Note:
Tears are unable to drain down the
lacrimal punctum as it is turned away
from the eye.
They therefore pool and spill over the
lid margin.

Fig. 6.2 Ectropion – leading to stenosis of the lacrimal punctum and keratinization of the conjunctival surface.

Mucocele (see p. 169)
Blepharitis (see p. 143)
Blockage of nasolacrimal duct (see Fig. 6.3).

1. Assume nasolacrimal duct blockage if watering occurs in the absence of any lid or eye pathology.
2. Instill a drop of fluorescein into each eye – this should drain away within 5 minutes if the tear ducts are working adequately.
3. Wash out the lacrimal sac and duct – only attempt this if you have the correct equipment and are confident about the anatomy
   - drop of proxymetacaine 0.5% into **both** eyes – more comfortable for patient
   - identify lacrimal punctum and dilate with a punctum dilator (Fig. 6.5a)
   - use a 2 ml syringe filled with normal saline and fitted with a lacrimal cannula
   - insert cannula gently into the lower punctum and guide it through into the lacrimal sac – if there is an obstruction in the canaliculus (the duct connecting the punctal opening to the lacrimal sac near the nose) a spongy resistance will be felt (Fig. 6.5b)

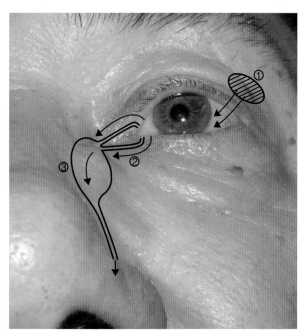

1. tears produced by lacrimal gland
2. flow across eye and drain into both upper (30%) and lower
   (70%) canaliculi
3. drain into lacrimal sac, then into nasal cavity

Fig. 6.3a   Normal production and drainage of tears.

- DO NOT FORCE the cannula through – an easy passage with a solid stop indicates that the cannula is pressing against the bone on the nasal side of the sac
- gently inject saline
- ask patient if they can taste the saline – if yes – then there is a patent system
- reflux through the upper lid punctum indicates blockage (Fig. 6.3b).

Referral

- routine to ophthalmology outpatients – only required if symptoms are significant and patient is willing to undergo surgery if required (dacryocystorhinostomy).

DRY EYE

1. Hypromellose 0.3% drops or Viscotears liquid gel four times daily.
2. Lacri-Lube ointment at night or three times daily in severe cases.

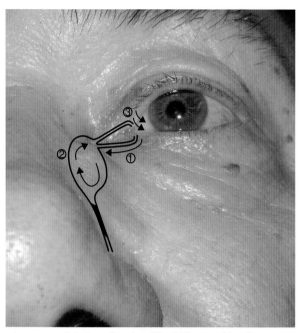

1. sac wash out – saline (see Fig. 6.5) passed into lower canaliculus
2. enters sac but cannot exit into nasal cavity
3. refluxes through upper punctum

Note: non-draining sac can become infected leading to dacryocystitis (Fig. 9.28)

Fig. 6.3b Site of NLD stenosis.

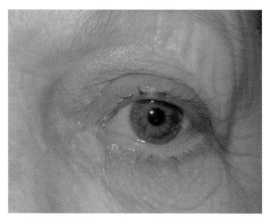

Fig. 6.4 Mucocele – typical position – compression may result in mucopus being refluxed into the tear film.

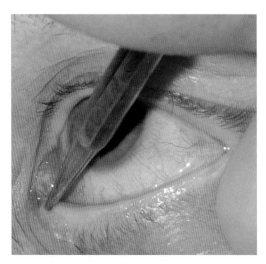

Fig. 6.5a Identify lacrimal punctum and dilate with a punctum dilator.

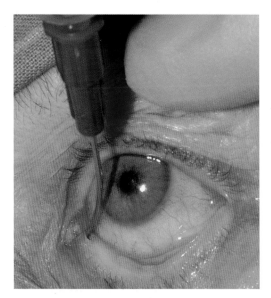

Fig. 6.5b Insert cannula gently into the lower punctum and guide it through into the lacrimal sac – if there is an obstruction in the canaliculus a spongy resistance will be felt.

Referral

- routine ophthalmology OPD if corneal staining persists despite above treatment – otherwise not required.

MANAGEMENT AND REFERRAL – CHILD

Failure of Canalization of Nasolacrimal Duct

Features
- chronic watering – often unilateral having initially been bilateral occasionally with purulent discharge
- 90% will resolve spontaneously by one year of age – 99% by two.

Management
1. Reassure parents – given that the condition usually resolves as above.
2. Keep the eye clean by gently washing away encrusted debris.
3. Massage the lacrimal sac – with forefinger, gently massage downwards from the corner of the eye halfway down the side of the nose, ten times, three times daily.

Referral
- ophthalmology outpatients soon (non-urgent) even if over 12 months of age
- if marked infection and discharge refer to ophthalmologist within 24 hours – beware of orbital cellulitis if there is surrounding erythema (see p. 147–149).

Suspected Congenital Glaucoma

Features
- big eyes – 'beautiful big eyes'
- watering
- parental concern with vision
- cloudy cornea.

Referral
- ophthalmologist within 24 hours.

Chapter 7

Contact Lens Problems

- common and usually related to overwear or poor hygiene
- patient usually gives an accurate history and diagnosis is rarely a problem
- assess whether acute or chronic.

ACUTE PROBLEMS

CHRONIC PROBLEMS

CONTACT LENS OVERWEAR

Features

- acutely red painful eye, with watery 'discharge' – often bilateral
- common – usually from wearing lenses overnight.

Management

1. Confirm that contact lenses have been removed by the patient.
2. Instill a drop of topical anesthetic into each eye to allow examination.
3. Stain the cornea with fluorescein – a diffuse pattern of staining is common centrally.
4. Look for a corneal ulcer and if present treat and refer appropriately (see p. 38).
5. Instill a drop of cyclopentolate 1% (Mydrilate) to dilate the pupil and relieve painful ciliary muscle spasm if light is painful (photophobia).

6. Wear dark glasses for 1–2 days if photophobic.
7. Instil chloramphenicol ointment 1%.
8. Patch the eye – or the worst eye if both eyes involved with a double pad (Figs 9.13, 9.14) for 24 hours.
9. Contact lenses should not be reinserted until checked by optician.

Referral and Follow Up

- **corneal ulcer.** Immediately to ophthalmologist
- **punctate corneal staining only.** No follow up required – review by optician before inserting contact lenses again.

ACCIDENTAL INSTILLATION OF LENS CLEANING SOLUTION

Features

- usually unilateral but may be bilateral – acute pain with watery 'discharge'.

Management

1. Instill a drop of topical anesthetic to allow examination.
2. Ensure from history that contact lenses have been removed.
3. Remove the lenses if still in eye – use a drop of fluorescein to help identify the lens.
4. Irrigate the eye either using a free running drip set connected to a 1 liter bag of normal saline with the patient lying down or use sterile water.
5. If the lenses have already been previously removed by the patient for more than one hour irrigation is unnecessary.
6. Stain with fluorescein if not already used – diffuse punctate staining is usually present and indicates chemical damage – treat as an abrasion (see p. 24) and patch the worst eye if bilateral.
7. Look for a corneal ulcer and treat appropriately (see p. 38).
8. In severe cases instill a drop of cylopentolate 1% to relieve pain due to iris muscle spasm.
9. Discharge on chloramphenicol 1% ointment four times daily for 5 days.
10. Instruct patient to leave out contact lenses until they have been checked for embedded foreign bodies by their optician, and not to reinsert them for a minimum of 1 week.

Referral and Follow Up

- corneal ulcer. Immediately to the ophthalmologist
- severe corneal staining with fluorescein. Review after 24 hours and if no improvement refer to ophthalmologist
- mild unilateral or bilateral corneal staining. Not required
- advise the patient to attend optician as in 10. above if appropriate.

INTOLERANCE TO CONTACT LENS WEAR

Features

- may occur after years of trouble-free wear
- may be exacerbated by change in style of lens such as hard to soft, or change of cleaning solution
- may present as chronic ocular irritation.

Management

1. Remove contact lenses if in situ.
2. Evert the upper lid (Figs 2.25–2.28) – a red irregular undersurface usually indicates a chronic allergic response.
3. Stain the cornea with fluorescein – diffuse staining may be present with dirty or poorly fitting lenses.
4. Look for a corneal ulcer – this appears as a solid staining area – if present treat and refer appropriately (see p. 38).
5. Advise patient not to reinsert lenses until they have been examined by their optician – adjustment of lens type or fitting or can then be assessed.
6. If corneal staining with fluorescein is present and provided there is no evidence of corneal ulceration – treat with chloramphenicol 1% four times daily for one week.

Referral and Follow Up

- corneal ulcer. Immediately to the ophthalmologist
- severe corneal staining with fluorescein. Review after 24 hours and if no improvement refer to ophthalmologist
- mild unilateral or bilateral corneal staining. Not required – but should see optician prior to reusing lenses.

LOST CONTACT LENS

Features

- can occur spontaneously or more typically after sport
- soft lenses may cause few symptoms despite being folded under the upper lid.

Management

1. Instill a drop of topical anesthetic to enable examination.
2. Check from the history that the patient has not in fact removed the lens.
3. Examine with a slit lamp if available, otherwise under a good light and look in the lower conjunctival fornix – the gutter between the lower eyelid and the globe – by making the patient look up whilst you pull their lower lid down (Fig. 2.32).

4. Ask them to look left and right whilst looking up, and look for the lens in the folds of conjunctiva.
5. Evert the upper lid (Figs 2.25–2.28) by:
   - asking the patient to look down, and keep looking down
   - place the wooden stick of a cotton bud horizontally across the mid portion of the upper lid, grasp their eyelashes firmly and gently rotate the lid upwards over the stick
   - remove the stick and hold the eyelid in position by holding the lashes against the brow
   - make the patient look left and right in downgaze
   - place the cotton bud under the upper lid into the upper conjunctival fornix and sweep it once - this is uncomfortable. Soak the cotton bud in local anesthetic first.
6. If the lens is still not found instill fluorescein which may help identify the lens and observe under a blue light – if the patient has soft lenses advise them before instilling the drop that this will stain the lens.
7. Repeat steps 3 to 5 if required.
8. If the lens is found ensure that it is intact – if part is missing search for this (Fig. 2.31).
9. Discharge on chloramphenicol ointment 1% four times daily for one week and advise patient not to reinsert contact lenses for this period.
10. Patch the eye for 24 hours if an abrasion is present.

Referral and Follow Up

- only required if lens is not found or part is missing – refer to the ophthalmologist within 24 hours after instilling chloramphenicol ointment and padding the eye
- if severe abrasion present but lens is found, treat abrasion (see p. 24).

CORNEAL ULCER FOLLOWING CONTACT LENS WEAR

- this usually occurs with soft or disposable lens wear and is fully discussed under 'corneal ulcers' on page 38.

Chapter 8

Lids

Common Complaints

Less Common

IRRITATION

Two main causes both of which are usually chronic with acute exacerbations.

1. **Blepharitis.** Crusted or matted eyelashes often with injected thickened lid margins and chronic itch (Fig. 8.1).
2. **Allergy.** Often atopic patients with eczema or secondary to eye drops (Fig. 8.2).

BLEPHARITIS

- extremely common, chronic, bilateral lid and eye irritation
- irritation rather than pain
- acute on chronic exacerbations common
- often associated with tear film deficiency.

Management

1. Advise that the condition is chronic and although treatment may relieve symptoms it will not cure the underlying problem.

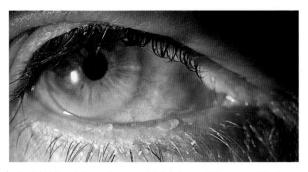

Fig. 8.1   Blepharitis – injected crusted lids often with matted lashes

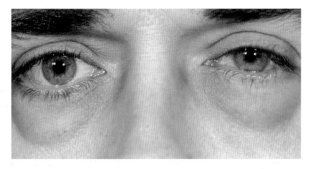

Fig. 8.2   Allergy – edematous lids and mildly injected eye – watering is common – a purulent discharge would be typical of conjunctivitis (see p. 51)

2. Lid hygiene – clean the lid margins thoroughly morning and night by
   - pulling the skin of the outer lid margins laterally to put the lid margin under tension
   - use a clean lint cloth or flannel dampened with either a mild solution of saline – one teaspoon of salt in a tumbler of cooled boiled water – or mild solution of baby shampoo
   - firmly rub the margins to remove grease and debris associated with the condition – keeping the eye shut
   - this treatment should be continued indefinitely.
3. If the lids are very injected start on Fucithalmic ointment 1% twice daily firmly rubbed into the eyelid margins at the base of their eyelashes for 3 weeks – there is no need to instill this into the eye.
4. Stain the cornea with fluorescein and observe under a blue light for a marginal ulcer (see p. 39).

Referral and Follow Up

- not required in the absence of corneal pathology
- if corneal staining is present refer to ophthalmologist within 24–48 hours.

ALLERGY

- acute or chronic
- common allergens include housedust, fur, feathers, antibiotic eye drops, makeup or contact lens solution
- may be more marked in atopic individuals.

Management

1. If diffuse inflammation is present, treat as periorbital cellulitis (see p. 147).
2. Swollen, edematous but not inflamed lids and periorbital tissue are typical findings in an acute allergic response.
3. Conjunctiva may be similarly swollen and appears as a pale yellow colored bag of fluid surrounding the cornea and even hanging over the lid margin (Fig. 2.7b).
4. Cold compresses – soak a clean flannel in cold water and place over the closed eyes or use crushed ice if available.
5. Identify any possible allergen from the history such as grass pollen, feather pillows, debris from sand pit with children.
6. Stop any antibiotic eye drops, and do not substitute another.
7. If contact lenses are worn remove and leave out until reviewed – see referral below.
8. Stop using eye makeup until condition has resolved then change to a hypoallergenic variety.
9. Otrivine-Antistin eye drops three times daily or Opatanol (olopatadine) drops twice daily – but be aware that any eye drops may exacerbate the problem.

Referral and Follow Up

1. Suspected cellulitis
   - children – admit under pediatricians
   - adults – discuss with ophthalmologist and start on treatment (see p. 147–149).
2. Eye drop or contact lens related – ophthalmologist within 24 hours.
3. Other allergens – discharge on above treatment and advise to return if no improvement within 24 hours.

INFECTION

Lid infection may be:

- localized – stye, blepharitis, infected chalazion
- diffuse – preseptal or orbital cellulitis (Fig. 8.4a,b).

LOCALIZED INFECTION

- **stye** – this is centered around an eyelash and may have a pointing head visible
- **infected chalazion** – an injected lump within the body of the lid – a previous longstanding painless lump may have been present prior to infection (Fig. 3.1).

Management

1. Document the visual acuity in each eye.
2. If a stye – pull out the eyelashes involved as this helps to drain the small abscess and discharge on chloramphenicol 1% drops four times daily for 10 days.
3. Recurrent stye – check urine for diabetes and treat or refer as appropriate.
4. Infected chalazion – start on systemic antibiotics such as oral Magnapen 500 mg four times daily for 10 days in addition to chloramphenicol 1% drops four times daily.
5. Incision of cyst (Figs 9.5–9.14).

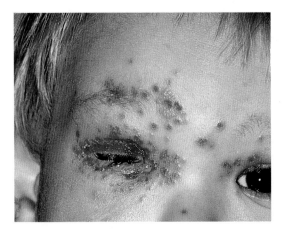

Fig. 8.3 If an initially localized infection spreads to the rest of the eyelid in a child, then treat as periorbital cellulitis (see p. 147).

Referral and Follow Up

- not required unless infection fails to resolve or worsens
- warn parents of children to return immediately if there are signs of spread or systemic illness
- if a residual cyst remains following resolution of an infected chalazion refer routinely to ophthalmology outpatients only if the patient wishes surgery – otherwise discharge.

DIFFUSE INFECTION

- diffuse erythema and infection may follow localized infection rapidly leading to preseptal (superficial tissue) or orbital (deep tissue) cellulitis (Fig. 8.4)
- the latter may be life threatening if not treated promptly.

Ask Directly

Trauma

- scratches, insect bites and plucked eyebrows can be the origin sites of infection.

History of Styes, Lid Infections, Sinusitis or Upper Respiratory Tract Infection

- orbital tissue may become involved from adjacent infected regions (Figs 8.5, 8.6) and particularly from the ethmoid sinuses in children.

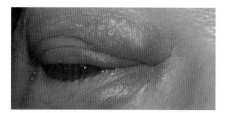

Fig. 8.4a,b Orbital cellulitis – note gross conjunctival swelling – eye movements may be restricted.

a

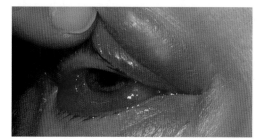

b

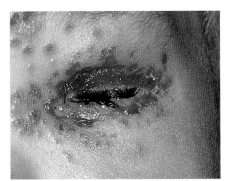

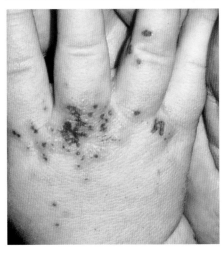

Figs 8.5, 8.6   Primary herpes simplex infection – lesions on hand transferred from rubbing eye. Fig. 8.5 (top) reproduced with permission from Kanski J J, 2003, Clinical Ophthalmology: A Systemic Approach, Butterworth–Heinemann.

Malaise
■ particularly important in children who may rapidly develop systemic symptoms.

Examination

1. Document visual acuity in each eye.
2. Look for source of infection such as stye, scratch or plucked eyebrows.
3. Check eye movements – restriction leads to double vision and indicates orbital cellulitis.
4. Test for double vision using a target at least 2 feet from the patient – if you get too close you will induce physiological (normal) double vision.
5. Painful restricted movement occurs in orbital cellulitis and the eye itself may be red and chemotic (Fig. 8.4b).

6. Check and document pupil reactions – an afferent pupil defect (see p. 7) may occur in orbital cellulitis secondary to optic nerve compression.

Management and Referral

Children

1. Children should be admitted immediately for systemic antibiotics under the pediatricians.
2. Give intravenous systemic antibiotics after discussing with pediatricians if a delay is likely.
3. Arrange for an MRI or CT of head, sinuses and orbits.

Adults

1. If diplopia (double vision), decreased vision or afferent pupil defect is present admit immediately under the ophthalmologists for intravenous antibiotics.
2. Arrange head, sinus and orbital CT or MRI.
3. If there are no systemic or ocular features other than lid involvement in an adult, treat with oral antibiotics such as oral Magnapen 500 mg four times daily and refer to the ophthalmologist within 24 hours.
4. X-ray orbit if there is a history of sinusitis or previous trauma.

SHINGLES

- skin vesicles with subsequent crusting in herpes zoster ophthalmicus (HZO) may be mild (Fig. 2.39) or very severe with scarring (Fig. 8.7)
- involvement of the eye does not always occur even if the lids are involved.

Management

If eye is red or vision reduced see 'Red Eye' – shingles, page 43. For **normal underlying eye:**

1. Treat skin with emollient cream (E45) to prevent crusting.
2. Start Shingles pack – 800 mg Zovirax orally five times daily for 1 week.
3. Analgesia orally or parenteral as the pain may be excruciating.
4. Neuralgia is common following shingles – the following may be effective if simple analgesia fails:
   - transcutaneous nerve stimulation (TENS) – see 'referral' below
   - amitriptyline – 25 mg once daily orally as a starting dose – beware urinary retention and cardiotoxicity
   - carbamazepine 100 mg at night orally – narrow therapeutic range and need to monitor full blood count.
5. Corneal anesthesia may occur – check by rolling a soft tissue corner to a point and gently touching the cornea – approach the eye from the side, not the front, or patient will see you approaching and blink.

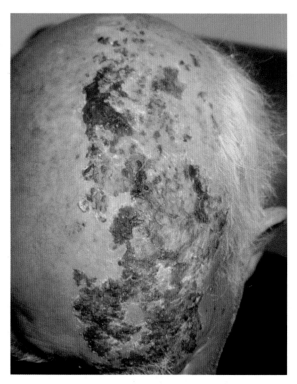

Fig. 8.7 Severe scab formation in shingles.

Referral

- in the absence of eye signs or symptoms no referral is required – but advise patient to reattend if eye symptoms subsequently develop
- red eye – ophthalmologist within 24 hours – iritis and dendritiform ulcers are common
- corneal anesthesia – discuss with ophthalmologist within 24 hours
- neuralgia
    obtain advice from physicians prior to starting amitriptyline or carbamazepine
    physiotherapy outpatient appointment for TENS
    if persistent and severe refer to neurologist or pain clinic if available.

ECTROPION (Fig. 8.8)

- lower lid turned out with inner surface exposed
- watering eye common as lacrimal punctum is turned away from eye (Fig. 8.8)

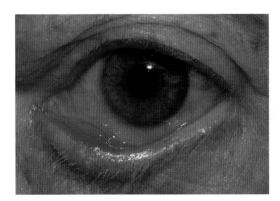

Fig. 8.8 Ectropion – the lower lid is turned out from the ocular surface – in this case by general laxity of the lower lid tissues – senile ectropion.

■ common in elderly due to lax tissues but can occur after facial burns and with chronic skin conditions – cicatricial ectropion.

Management and Referral

1. Stain the cornea with fluorescein and look for diffuse fine staining indicating corneal exposure.
2. GelTears four times during the day, Lacri-Lube ointment at night (blurs vision).
3. Ophthalmology outpatients routinely.

ENTROPION AND INGROWING LASHES (TRICHIASIS)
(Fig. 8.9)

■ **entropion** – lid has turned in on itself allowing eyelashes to touch the eye
■ **trichiasis** – ingrowing, aberrant eyelashes – can occur without entropion.

Management and Referral

1. Trichiasis – epilate (pull out) the offending lashes with forceps.
2. Entropion – use Steristrips or Sellotape as a temporary measure to pull the lower lid off the globe – to do this (Fig. 2.30):
    ■ dry the skin
    ■ place one end of a Steristrip on the skin just below the lashes
    ■ pull down gently until lashes are pulled off the globe
    ■ stick other end onto cheek
    ■ use three Steristrips in a row.
3. Stain the cornea with dilute fluorescein and look for lash-induced abrasions.

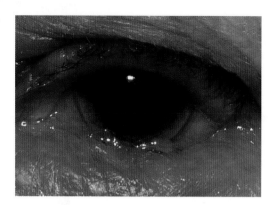

Fig. 8.9 Entropion – the lid is turned towards the eye – the lashes are in contact with the ocular surface – can occur in both the lower and upper lid

4. If corneal staining is present prescribe chloramphenicol ointment 1% three times daily for 5 days.
5. Refer to ophthalmologist for definitive surgery.

Chapter 9

Tumors of the Eye and Surrounding Tissues

EYELIDS

Cysts and other lumps

Most are benign – features suggestive of malignancy include:

- ill-defined edge
- relentless increase in size
- bleeding, crusting, change in color
- loss of lashes.

BENIGN LESIONS

Chalazion (Figs 9.1, 9.2, 9.3)

- common, recurrent on both upper and lower lids
- non-tender, firm, rounded lump
- associated with blepharitis (see p. 60, 143)
- if infected may lead to periorbital cellulitis (see p. 147)
- main swelling is above lash line – higher than that of a stye (Fig. 9.3)
- consider sebaceous cell carcinoma if recurrent – especially in the elderly.

Management and referral
1. Conservative initially – many will resolve spontaneously with
   - chloramphenicol four times daily if infected
   - firm massage with a warm flannel three times daily.

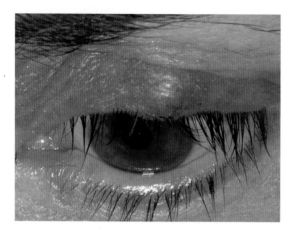

Fig. 9.1 Typical chalazion or meibomian cyst – the cyst is in the body of the lid but may extend to the lid margin.

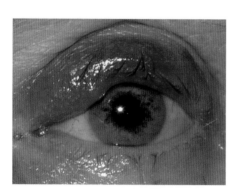

Fig. 9.2 Infected chalazion – may be difficult to see the lesion itself if the lid is swollen – but can be identified by palpation.

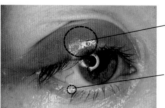

Chalazion – typical position in body of either upper or lower lid

Typical position of stye is at the base of an eyelash on the lid margin

Fig. 9.3 Lid showing position of stye, chalazion, lashes, etc. Reproduced with permission from Kanski J J, 2003, Clinical Ophthalmology: A Systemic Approach, Butterworth–Heinemann.

2. Surgical incision and curettage – if patient wishes removal soon, unsightly, or fails to resolve over 2–3 months. Treat any infection prior to surgery.
3. Children – conservative treatment, surgery only if large or recurrent as general anesthesia required.

Incision and Curettage (I & C) (Figs 9.4–9.14)

- only if unsightly or repeated episodes of infection
- if patient complains of irritation – particularly if a contact lens wearer
- child – only if large as may result in amblyopia from pressure on eye – **otherwise leave** as if lesion is small, and visual acuity normal removal under general anesthetic is unjustified
- if small and little bother, reassure and discharge – spontaneous resolution may occur.

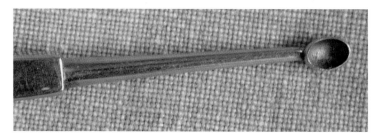

Fig. 9.4 Curette used to remove cyst contents.

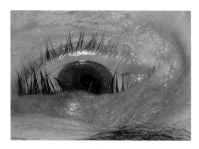

Fig. 9.5 Lie the patient flat – put topical anesthetic into each eye.

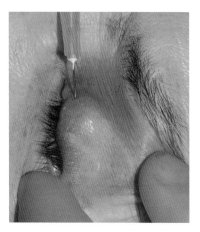

Fig. 9.6 Inject local anesthetic into lid – around the cyst and massage in.

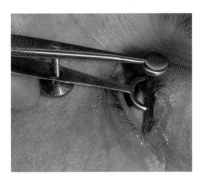

Fig. 9.7 Place chalazion clamp centrally over cyst as shown.

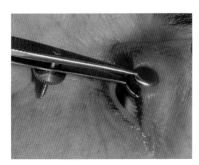

Fig. 9.8 Tighten the clamp – provides protection, good grip and hemostasis.

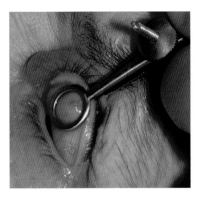

Fig. 9.9 Evert the lid with the clamp – if it slips, reposition and tighten.

Stye

■ common acute small abscess around the base of an eyelash.

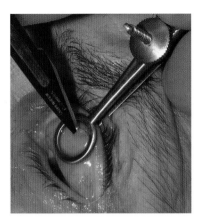

Fig. 9.10 Incise the cyst at right angles to the lid margin – do not cut into the lid margin itself.

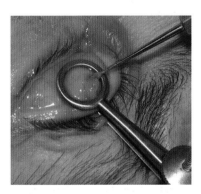

Fig. 9.11 Scoop out the cyst contents – wipe away with a gauze swab.

Management and Referral
1. Pull out the lash.
2. Chloramphenicol drops or ointment four times daily for 5 days.
3. Refer to ophthalmologist if failure to start resolving within 48 hours in children – they are at higher risk of periorbital cellulitis (see p. 147).

Papilloma and Skin Tags (Figs 9.15, 9.16)

- often at the lid margin – may be flat or pedunculated with a craggy surface
- often present for years.

Management and Referral
1. Not required if no evidence of malignancy (see p. 153) and patient unconcerned.
2. If not involving the eyelashes

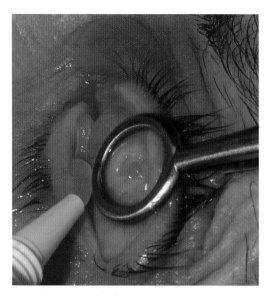

Fig. 9.12 Instill chloramphenicol ointment – note the empty cyst sac.

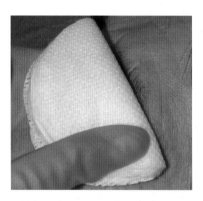

Fig. 9.13 Return lid to normal position, remove clamp, place eye pad folded in half and apply pressure.

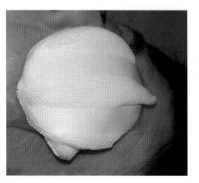

Fig. 9.14 Place further eye pad over folded pad and tape down to apply pressure.

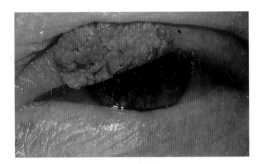

Fig. 9.15 Sessile papilloma – note broad base but typical craggy surface.

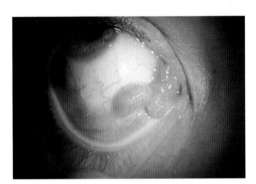

Fig. 9.16 Pedunculated papilloma involving conjunctiva. Reproduced with permission from Kanski J J, 2003, Clinical Ophthalmology: A Systemic Approach, Butterworth–Heinemann.

- can be removed with cautery under local anesthetic
- refer routinely to the ophthalmologist if on lash line.

Cyst of Moll (Fig. 9.17)

- small, clear cyst on lid margin.

Management and Referral
1. cysts can be drained by
   - proxymetacaine 0.5% local anesthetic into eye – helps reduce blink reflex
   - incise and de-roof with an orange needle mounted on a 2 ml syringe to act as a handle
   - do not attempt this near the inferior canaliculus (medial end of lower lid) as you can damage tear drainage system
   - referral unnecessary but recurrence common.

Solar and Seborrheic Keratosis (Fig. 9.18)

- sun-damaged skin often with elevated lesions.

Management and Referral
1. No intervention or referral required unless recent change in lesion.

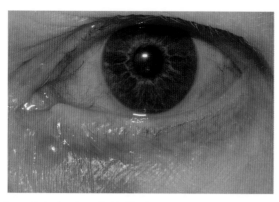

Fig. 9.17 Cyst of Moll – clear fluid-filled cyst near the lid margin.

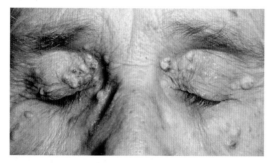

Fig. 9.18 Sebaceous cysts and actinic damage are usually longstanding.

In General
- if patient is undecided about surgery and lesion benign – discharge
- do not attempt surgery on children or young adults.

MALIGNANT LESIONS

Basal Cell Carcinoma (Fig. 9.19a, b)

- pearly edged 'ulcer' usually on lower lid with a central crater that may bleed and crust over
- may appear as a discrete nodule or as a diffuse nodular mass usually on the lid margin
- slow relentless growth over months.

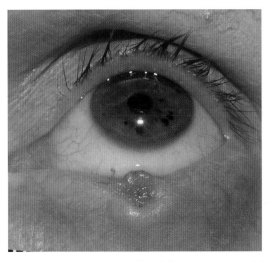

Fig. 9.19a   Basal cell carcinoma – typical nodular appearance with central crater and pearly edge. Note presence of iris freckles.

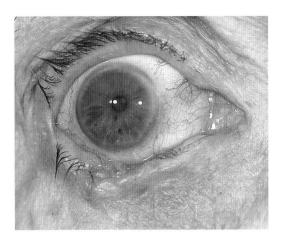

Fig. 9.19b   Diffuse basal cell carcinoma – note destruction of eyelashes.

Squamous Cell Carcinoma (Fig. 9.20)

- may be similar in appearance and site to a basal cell carcinoma
- growth may be rapid over a few weeks
- may originate in longstanding solar keratosis (Fig. 9.18).

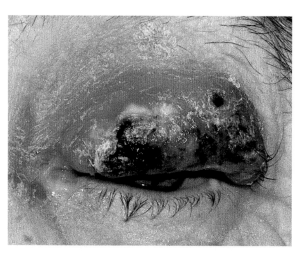

Fig. 9.20 Squamous cell carcinoma – diffuse lesion with rapid destructive growth – regional lymph nodes were already involved.

Malignant Melanoma (Fig. 9.21a,b,c)

- usually pigmented often arising from a longstanding nevus
- malignancy indicated by change in size, color or bleeding.

Sebaceous Cell Carcinoma

- usually in the elderly and may mimic chronic blepharitis or recurrent chalazion.

Management and Referral

All lesions suspected of malignancy require referral to ophthalmologist for biopsy.

EYE – SURFACE

Conjunctival Lesions

The conjunctiva is a membrane that covers the 'white' of the eye as well as the inner surface of the eyelids (Figs 1.1, 9.22).

Pigmented

- usually simple nevi or malignant melanoma
- growth, bleeding or change in color indicate possible malignancy
- benign nevi may enlarge at puberty or during pregnancy.

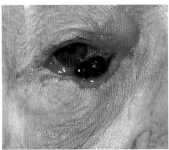

a

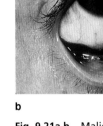

b

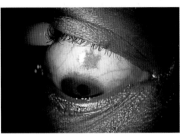

c

Fig. 9.21a,b Malignant melanoma. In **b** the presentation may be late as the lesion is hidden in the lower fornix.
Fig. 9.21c Conjunctival melanosis.

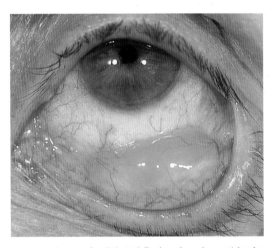

Fig. 9.22 Conjunctival cyst. If solid and flesh colored, consider lymphoma – typically bilateral.

Management and Referral
1. If longstanding and unchanged – discharge.
2. If evidence of malignancy refer to ophthalmologist for biopsy.

Non-pigmented (Fig. 9.23)

Pterygium
- extends across the corneal surface
- usually on the nasal side
- associated with living in hot dry climates.

Management and Referral
1. If asymptomatic and lesion is not near pupil margin – discharge.
2. If recurrent inflammation or encroaching upon pupil – refer ophthalmologist.
3. If acutely inflamed
   - Predsol or Betnesol drops three times daily PROVIDED there is no evidence of herpetic ulceration (see p. 38).

Conjunctival Cyst (Figs 9.22, 9.24)
- transparent
- usually asymptomatic.

Management and Referral
1. If asymptomatic – no intervention and discharge.
2. Large or symptomatic
   - topical proxymetacaine 0.5% both eyes
   - using an orange needle on a 2 ml syringe as a handle, incise cyst
   - topical chloramphenicol three times daily for 5 days.
3. High recurrence rate unless 'de-roofed'.

Conjunctival Chemosis
- not a lesion but reactive edema (Fig. 2.7b)
- usually allergic response
- occasionally secondary to thyroid dysfunction.

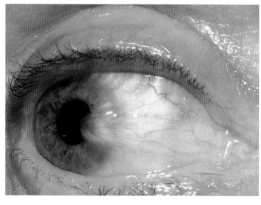

Fig. 9.23 Pterygium – may be stable for many years – requires removal if threatens visual axis.

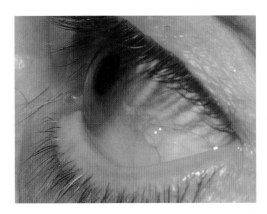

Fig. 9.24 Conjunctival cyst – longstanding and frequently asymptomatic.

Management and Referral
See p. 145.

Red, Painful or Irritable Lesions

- if at the edge of the cornea (limbus) these are usually foci of inflammation or ulcers rather than tumors (Figs 2.34, 2.35)
- nodular episcleritis (Fig. 2.38a) may present as a red edematous lump near the limbus – usually at 3 or 9 o'clock.

Management and Referral
1. Stain with fluorescein which will highlight a foreign body (see p. 27), abrasion (see p. 24) or ulcer (see p. 38).
2. If painful and not due to a foreign body, abrasion or ulcer refer to ophthalmologist within 24 hours.
3. If very painful (possible scleritis, see p. 41) discuss immediately.

INTERNAL OCULAR TUMORS

iris – pigmented and non-pigmented   p. 165
retina and choroid   p. 166

IRIS

Pigmented Lesions

- if small multiple and longstanding these are usually iris freckles (Fig. 9.19a)
- if single, larger than about 1 mm, or distorting the pupil – consider melanoma.

Management and Referral

1. Longstanding iris freckles require no intervention – reassure and discharge.
2. If any increase in number or size of freckles, or any suspicion of malignancy, refer to ophthalmology outpatients – melanomas of the iris do not invariably require excision.

Non-pigmented Lesions

- cysts can occur after surgery – months to years
- amelanotic melanomas are very rare.

Management and Referral

1. Routinely to the ophthalmology outpatients.
2. If any suspicion of malignancy – growth, change in color or pupil distortion – refer to ophthalmologist soon.

RETINA AND CHOROID

Choroidal Nevus (Fig. 9.25)

- usually incidental finding
- may be slightly raised with overlying yellow deposits – drusen
- can be large.

Choroidal Melanoma

- usually presents with decreased vision or 'shadowing' in the visual field

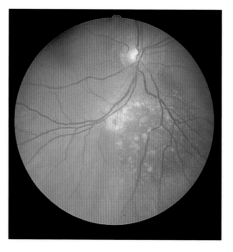

Fig. 9.25 Choroidal nevus – note overlying drusen.

- may present with secondary glaucoma or hemorrhage within the eye
- most common primary internal ocular tumor in adults
- dark elevated fixed mass either near the front of the eye – ciliary body tumor or further back towards the optic nerve
- localized large 'conjunctival' blood vessels (feeder vessels) often indicate an anterior underlying tumor
- retinal detachment or vitreous hemorrhage may overlie the tumor.

Management and Referral

1. Any pigmented fundal lesion greater than the diameter of the optic disc – ophthalmology outpatients.
2. If elevated or associated retinal detachment or vitreous bleed – discuss immediately with ophthalmologist.

Secondaries – Metastases

- most common internal ocular tumor overall
- rapid growth
- usually sited at the posterior pole – optic disc and macula
- often pale elevated lesions with poorly defined edges
- primary is usually breast in females, bronchus in males
- associated field defects may be present due to cerebral metastases.

Management and Referral

1. Investigate for the primary.
2. Refer to ophthalmologist within 48 hours.
3. Involve relevant specialty for investigation of possible primary.

Retinoblastoma

- most common primary intraocular tumor in children
- very rare
- may present with white pupil reflex – leucocoria – or squint.

Management and Referral

1. Ophthalmologist within 24 hours.
2. Siblings and both parents should be examined and given genetic counseling.

PERIORBITAL AND ORBITAL

Proptosis

The eye appears more prominent (Figs 9.26, 9.27)

- may indicate an underlying orbital or sinus tumor pushing the eye from behind
- consider dysthyroid eye disease which is far more common (see p. 53)

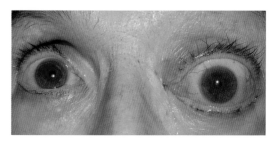

Fig. 9.26   Prominent left eye – orbital tumor pushing globe forward.

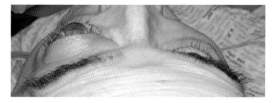

Fig. 9.27   Viewed from above – proptosis is clearly seen.

- orbital cellulitis – abscess behind eye (see p. 147)
- orbital pseudotumor – rare orbital inflammatory disease.

Management and Referral
1. Thyroid suspect (see p. 53).
2. Painless proptosis with normal visual acuity and pupils – refer to ophthalmologist within 24 hours.
3. All patients will require a CT or MRI scan of their orbital region.

LACRIMAL SAC LESIONS

The lacrimal sac lies between the nasal side of the eye and the bridge of the nose.

Abscess (Fig. 9.28)

- an abscess of this sac – dacryocystitis – can occur spontaneously or after a prolonged period of a watering eye – suggesting the tear drainage apparatus is blocked (Fig. 6.3b)
- frequently recurrent.

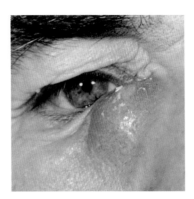

Fig. 9.28 Dacryocystitis – an abscess in the lacrimal sac – typical position.

Management and Referral
1. Oral Magnapen 500 mg for 10 days or any other broad spectrum antibiotic cover.
2. Refer to ophthalmologist within 24 hours.
3. Do not lance unless very distended and failing to respond to antibiotics – this may cause a fistula and detrimentally affect final outcome.

Non-inflamed, Non-tender Fluctuant Mass

- mucocele within the lacrimal sac
- associated with an ipsilateral watering eye
- mucopurulent discharge into eye if pressed firmly.

Management and Referral
1. Massage lesion to expel contents (Fig. 6.4).
2. Refer to ophthalmology outpatients routinely.

Chapter 10

Eye Surgery and Complications

Any pain, bleeding, or sudden change in vision following recent eye surgery of any type needs to be discussed with an ophthalmologist immediately.

CATARACT SURGERY

Main Techniques (Fig. 10.1)

1. **Phacoemulsification** – modern, small incision surgery.
2. **Extracapsular lens extraction** – older technique with large incision.

PHACOEMULSIFICATION

- method of choice in most developed countries
- usually under local anesthesia – eye drops alone can be used thus avoiding needles
- rapid visual recovery.

Basic Steps

- pupil is dilated to gain access to the cataract that lies behind the iris diaphragm
- small incision made into the side of the cornea – approximately 3 millimeters
- anterior surface membrane of cataract removed

Phacoemulsification cataract surgery

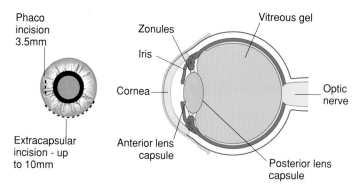

Phaco
incision
3.5mm

Zonules

Iris

Cornea

Vitreous gel

Optic
nerve

Extracapsular
incision - up
to 10mm

Anterior lens
capsule

Posterior lens
capsule

If the posterior capsule is broken - vitreous gel may prolapse through the wound. Less likely with small incision surgery.

The zonules support the lens capsule

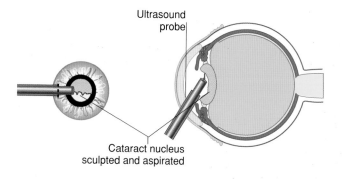

Ultrasound
probe

Cataract nucleus
sculpted and aspirated

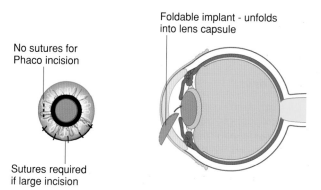

Foldable implant - unfolds
into lens capsule

No sutures for
Phaco incision

Sutures required
if large incision

Fig. 10.1 Cataract surgery.

- cataract emulsified and aspirated using an ultrasound probe
- foldable lens implant inserted through the wound into the correct plane
- wound is self sealing – sutures rarely required
- postoperative antibiotics and steroids (see p. 192).

EXTRACAPSULAR LENS EXTRACTION

- only rarely the treatment of choice in modern well equipped centers
- not suitable for topical anesthesia
- higher risk of postoperative astigmatism and intraoperative vitreous loss
- longer recovery period.

Basic Steps

- pupil dilated
- large incision at junction of clear cornea and sclera (limbus)
- anterior surface membrane of cataract incised
- cataract prolapsed out through wound
- lens implant inserted into correct plane
- wound sutured
- postoperative antibiotics and steroids (see p. 192).

COMPLICATIONS

Appearance of eye postoperatively depends upon the type of surgery and anesthesia.

Phacoemulsification

- eyes appear white and quiet after topical or general anesthesia
- if local anesthesia using a needle – periorbital bruising, conjunctival chemosis and hemorrhage possible.

Extracapsular

- large incision surgery – red eye common for up to 1 week regardless of anesthetic route

Immediate (0–2 days)

- discomfort or irritation is common for 24 to 48 hours and should settle
- pain may be secondary to an abrasion or raised intraocular pressure
- hazy vision is common in the first 24 hours
- wound dehiscence and iris prolapse – extracapsular technique only.

Early (2–7 days)

- increasing or non-resolving pain may be due to infection or raised intraocular pressure

- increasing injection, reduced acuity and loss of pupil red reflex (Fig. 1.12) may be due to infection or postoperative uveitis
- blurred vision – if present since operation which has neither deteriorated nor improved may be due to refractive error (need for glasses).

Late (7 days+)

- any persistent or worsening pain and redness, especially if associated with reduction in visual acuity should be considered as intraocular infection (Fig. 2.10)
- foreign body sensation – may be due to sutures – usually only with extracapsular technique as sutures rarely used in phacoemulsification technique (Fig. 10.2a)
- gradual blurring – due to membrane thickening behind implant – usually months to years after surgery (Fig. 4.15).

Management

1. Ensure patient is using postoperative eye drops as instructed (see p. 192).
2. Non-resolving pain, increasing pain, significant reduction in acuity, increasing injection – at any stage postoperatively – immediately refer to ophthalmologist as probable intraocular infection (endophthalmitis). The patient requires topical, intravitreal, and occasionally systemic antibiotics in addition to a vitrectomy and vitreous culture.
3. Initial discomfort only – reassure patient and review if fails to improve over 24–48 hours.

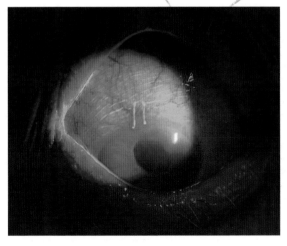

Fig. 10.2a   Loose sutures shown with fluorescein staining – these feel like a foreign body in the eye and require removal under slit lamp magnification.

4. Blurred vision – if stable without any dramatic reduction – may simply be due to need for glasses – test with a pinhole (see p. 5) vision will improve if this is the case – reassure and keep routine outpatient follow up.

Note

Patients may present as an emergency because they have been told that they 'have a cataract'.

1. Reassure – often all that is required – most patients will not know what a cataract is – they will not differentiate between cataract and cancer. A cataract is a loss in clarity of the normal lens within the eye – it is a normal change that occurs with increasing age, and more rarely following trauma or in association with systemic disease or drug treatment – if very mature it may lead to glaucoma or uveitis.
2. Ask – is vision a handicap or does it prevent normal daily activities – if not a handicap then surgery is not required.
3. Advise – cataract surgery is successful but NOT risk free – loss of the eye occurs in a very small number of cases – therefore patients with one eye or dense amblyopia need to be particularly cautious.

OCULOPLASTIC AND TRAUMA

The most common procedures are:

1. Ectropion or entropion repair.
2. Removal of eyelid cysts or tumors.
3. Reconstruction of lids if large lesion excised.
4. Traumatic lacerations.

Any problem following recent surgery for trauma to the eye itself needs to be immediately discussed with the ophthalmologist.

Complications

- wound dehiscence
- infection.

Management

Wound Dehiscence
1. Clean and treat with either chloramphenicol ointment or oral broad spectrum antibiotic if any sign of infection.
2. Remove any sutures that are abrading the surface of the eye.
3. Dress – Gelonet (vaseline gauze) and either eye pads or large sterile swabs.
4. Discuss with ophthalmologist and arrange review within 24 hours.

Infection
1. Clean and treat with chloramphenicol ointment if localized infection or oral broad spectrum antibiotic if any sign of more widespread cellulitis (see p. 146–149).
2. Discuss with ophthalmologist if no response or worse within 24 hours.
3. Any sign of wound infection in children should be treated aggressively (see p. 146–149) as rapid spread into frank periorbital cellulitis can occur.

LASER (EXCIMER) REFRACTIVE SURGERY

Excimer laser – disrupts molecular bonding and vaporizes tissue.

Two main techniques – both used in the correction of short sightedness (myopia) and less frequently for long sightedness (hypermetropia) or astigmatism.

Astigmatism simply describes a cornea that is more curved in one axis than the other – it has a surface contour shaped like a rugby ball as opposed to a football – which is spherical. It is not a disease, and is usually correctable with glasses or contact lenses. Progressive astigmatism may be associated with keratoconus (see p. 92). Reading glasses will be required for middle-aged patients postoperatively.

1. LASIK (Laser-assisted in situ keratomileusis).
2. PRK (Photo refractive keratectomy).

LASIK (Fig. 10.2b)

- the most common refractive surgical procedure

LASIK (laser-assisted in situ keratomileusis)

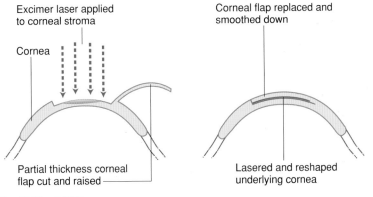

Excimer laser applied to corneal stroma

Cornea

Corneal flap replaced and smoothed down

Partial thickness corneal flap cut and raised

Lasered and reshaped underlying cornea

Fig. 10.2b LASIK.

- best technique for high refractive errors
- rapid visual recovery
- little or no postoperative discomfort.

Basic Steps

- extensive preoperative evaluation for suitability
- topical anesthetic drops
- partial thickness corneal flap with hinge cut using microkeratome cutter
- corneal flap folded back to expose underlying corneal tissue
- laser applied to exposed corneal surface
- corneal flap replaced
- topical antibiotics, steroids and lubricants.

Complications – Early and Late

- most complications are intraoperative and involve problems with the corneal flap, such as incomplete cut, 'button hole' (hole in the central part), or complete loss of flap – these complications are rare in the hands of experienced surgeons
- pain, watering and blurred vision
- overcorrection or regression
- infection and inflammation
- glare, haloes, dry eye.

Management

1. Adequate follow up should be central to competent management – all complications should present to the center which carried out the procedure, and **in all cases the operating surgeon or support staff should be contacted.**
2. Pain after LASIK is not normal – mild discomfort may last for up to 24 hours.
3. Ensure postoperative drops are being used.
4. Try to identify the corneal flap – a slit lamp is required for adequate examination – the flap may be displaced or, very rarely, missing – if the patient has been subject to trauma or rubbed their eye.
5. An abrasion may be present on the flap surface.
6. Other more subtle changes such as inflammation and growth of epithelial cells under the flap require a slit lamp examination.
7. Focal opacities – red eye and pain – indicate infection and should be treated as an ulcer (Fig. 2.33) – immediate referral to ophthalmologist required.

PRK

- used for low refractive errors
- often painful for 24 to 48 hours postoperatively
- longer recovery period.

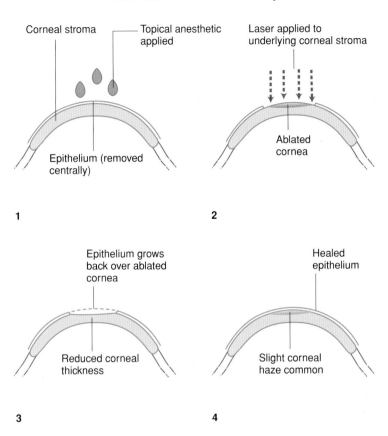

PRK Photo Refractive Keratectomy

Corneal stroma — Topical anesthetic applied — Laser applied to underlying corneal stroma

Epithelium (removed centrally) — Ablated cornea

1   **2**

Epithelium grows back over ablated cornea — Healed epithelium

Reduced corneal thickness — Slight corneal haze common

3   **4**

Fig. 10.2c   Photo refractive keratectomy.

Basic Steps (Fig. 10.2c)

- extensive preoperative evaluation for suitability
- topical anesthetic drops
- corneal epithelium removed
- laser applied to underlying corneal tissue
- topical antibiotics and steroids
- eye pads 24 hours.

Complications

Early

- pain – which may be severe as the epithelium heals – resolves within 48 hours

- blurred vision – may persist for 2 weeks or more
- infection – rare.

No flap created, therefore no flap complications.

Late
- glare, haloes, multiple images – all usually secondary to corneal scarring
- overcorrection or regression.

Management

1. Adequate follow up should be central to competent management – all complications should present to the center which carried out the procedure, and **in all cases the operating surgeon or support staff should be contacted.**
2. Ensure the patient is using the prescribed postoperative medication.
3. Persisting epithelial defect – treat as abrasion (see p. 24).
4. Corneal opacity – suspect an ulcer – (see p. 38, corneal ulcer).
5. Glare, haloes – usually late complication – refer to center or surgeon.

Note

Contraindications to laser refractive surgery include
- age – 21 is usually regarded as the lower limit
- systemic medications – particularly Roaccutane, steroids and recently started antidepressants
- active connective tissue disease
- pregnancy or breastfeeding
- any eye pathology – although not all cases are excluded
- very high refractive errors (–10 diopters and above) – may benefit from lens implant refractive surgery
- personality – high anxiety, obsessive or depressive.

SQUINT

- usually cosmetic – rarely to help manage double vision
- does not remove the need to wear glasses in children.

Basic Steps (Fig. 10.2d)

- usually carried out under general anesthesia – as most cases are children
- ocular motility assessment must reveal stable defect
- conjunctiva (mucous membrane covering the 'white' of the eye) is opened
- appropriate extraocular muscle identified as it attaches to the globe
- muscle either strengthened or weakened depending upon type of squint

Squint

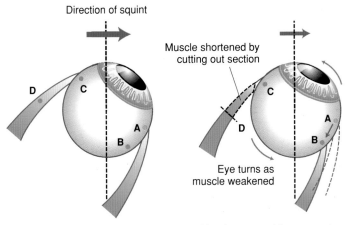

Direction of squint

Muscle shortened by cutting out section

Eye turns as muscle weakened

Muscle removed from normal insertion **A** and moved back to **B** weakens the action of the muscle. Eye moves as shown

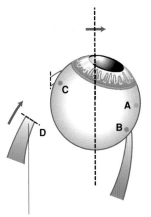

Straight

Muscle may have action strengthened by shortening and returning to original position

Muscle (now shortened) readvanced to original position

Fig. 10.2d   Squint surgery.

- to strengthen – muscle is usually shortened by excising a measured length, and then reattaching to its original site
- to weaken – it is detached, then reattached further back on the globe
- conjunctiva replaced and sutured
- topical drops or ointment as required (see p. 193)
- sutures do not require to be removed.

Complications

- pain
- infection
- double vision
- recurrence of squint.

Management

1. Pain is common for the first 24 hours and usually resolves with simple analgesia.
2. Persistent pain and irritation may be due to conjunctival sutures which can be trimmed or removed.
3. Infection should be treated with topical antibiotics as with conjunctivitis (see p. 51) – or if severe, systemically (see p. 147, cellulitis).
4. Double vision initially may resolve when swelling settles or adaptation to new eye position occurs.
5. Intractable double vision may occur if patient is unable to adapt to new eye position (this risk is usually ruled out preoperatively using prisms to mimic the effect of surgery) – refer back to surgeon, and patch one eye if required – as this will stop the diplopia.
6. Squint recurrence usually requires further surgery.

GLAUCOMA (TRABECULECTOMY)

- may present acutely (see p. 41) or more usually, as chronic glaucoma (see p. 95)
- most cases are successfully managed with topical medication (see p. 189, 195).

Basic Steps (Fig. 10.2e)

- surgery carried out if intraocular pressure control is unsatisfactory with topical medication
- may be under either local or general anesthesia
- the conjunctiva – usually in the superior aspect of the globe is incised and retracted
- a partial thickness trapdoor flap is cut and lifted in the underlying sclera – the hinge is along the junction with clear cornea
- a small full thickness block of sclera and trabecular meshwork (hence trabeculectomy) is removed from underneath the flap – making a fistula into the anterior chamber of the eye (in front of the iris, see p. 181)
- a small piece of iris is removed (iridectomy)
- the flap is replaced to cover the underlying fistula and sutured into place
- the conjunctiva is pulled back to cover the flap and sutured
- aqueous from the anterior chamber can then drain slowly under the flap and forms a fluid bubble at the surgical site (bleb).

Trabeculectomy

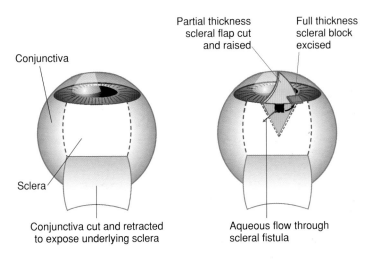

Partial thickness
scleral flap cut
and raised

Full thickness
scleral block
excised

Conjunctiva

Sclera

Conjunctiva cut and retracted
to expose underlying sclera

Aqueous flow through
scleral fistula

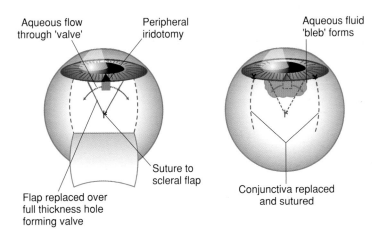

Aqueous flow
through 'valve'

Peripheral
iridotomy

Aqueous fluid
'bleb' forms

Suture to
scleral flap

Flap replaced over
full thickness hole
forming valve

Conjunctiva replaced
and sutured

note: a large conjunctival flap is not required but is shown here
for clarity

Fig. 10.2e Trabeculectomy.

Complications

- pain and reduced vision
- infection
- failure to reduce pressure or overdrainage with very low pressure.

Management

All patients must be referred to or discussed with the ophthalmologist in the early postoperative period.

1. Discomfort is common initially – usually settles within 1 week – ensure patient is compliant with prescribed treatment (see p. 192).
2. Blurred vision is common as the operation frequently changes the spectacle correction.
3. Infection should be treated aggressively – as intraocular spread can destroy the eye (endophthalmitis, Fig. 2.10).
4. Both overdrainage, which may result in a flat anterior chamber (Fig. 1.1), and underdrainage may require further surgery – a slit lamp and ability to measure intraocular pressure is required to accurately assess.

RETINAL DETACHMENT

- most common in myopes (short sighted)
- post traumatic
- may be preceded by floaters and flashes (Fig. 4.22)
- usually secondary to a retinal hole or tear, rarely secondary to an intraocular tumor
- if macula remains in place vision may be good.

Basic Steps (Fig. 10.2f)

1. Identify cause of detachment through dilated pupil.
2. Repair involves various techniques including:
    - aspiration of subretinal fluid through a scleral incision
    - cryotherapy to sclera overlying retinal defect – this helps the retina to 'stick' back
    - encircling band or buckle – these are placed on the sclera externally and indent the eye – pushing the sclera towards the retinal defect and removing traction which assists healing
    - laser – either applied through an internal probe – endolaser, or through an external lens.

Complications

- pain
- blurred vision
- redetachment.

Management

1. Pain is common postoperatively and usually settles within 48 hours on oral analgesia and prescribed topical medication (see p. 193).

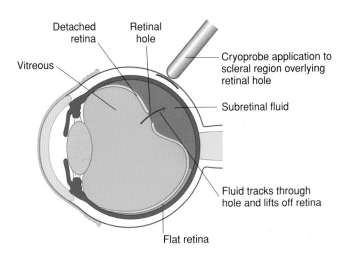

Retinal detachment

Detached retina

Retinal hole

Vitreous

Cryoprobe application to scleral region overlying retinal hole

Subretinal fluid

Fluid tracks through hole and lifts off retina

Flat retina

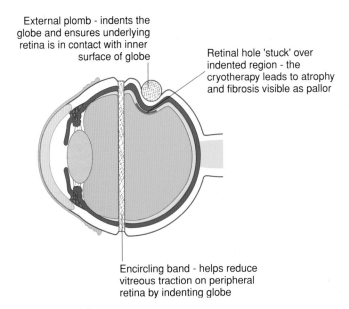

External plomb - indents the globe and ensures underlying retina is in contact with inner surface of globe

Retinal hole 'stuck' over indented region - the cryotherapy leads to atrophy and fibrosis visible as pallor

Encircling band - helps reduce vitreous traction on peripheral retina by indenting globe

Fig. 10.2f Retinal detachment.

2. Late-onset pain – weeks or months after surgery may be from a band or buckle migrating through the conjunctiva – refer to ophthalmologist within 24 hours. A protruding band or buckle may sometimes be

removed with forceps under topical anesthesia – however if soon after surgery, there is a risk of redetachment.

3. Blurred vision is common immediately postoperatively – final acuity depends upon the function of the macula postoperatively. If the macula was still in place before surgery (a 'macula on' detachment) then the visual prognosis is usually better than if the macula was detached – referral not required if there has not been a sudden postoperative deterioration and if within a week of surgery.

4. Sudden onset of blurred vision after surgery may indicate redetachment – discuss with and refer back to ophthalmologist.

LASER TREATMENT

- laser refractive surgery (LASIK or PRK) as above (see p. 175)
- diabetics
- glaucoma
- cataract.

1. **Argon** and **diode** laser – thermal burns.
2. **YAG** laser – delivers energy pulse in focused plane and disrupts tissue – non thermal.

Diabetics

1. Argon laser is used to ablate the retina to treat neovascular (proliferative) disease (PRP – pan retinal photocoagulation, Fig. 10.3) or more localized leaking vessels (focal laser).
2. Treatment is carried out on a slit lamp usually in several stages.
3. Discomfort is usually secondary to the bright laser flash rather than the small thermal retinal burn.
4. Outpatient procedure in most cases.

Glaucoma

1. YAG laser may be used to create a peripheral iridotomy (PI) in the iris in acute glaucoma.
2. This procedure creates a small hole in the peripheral iris, allowing aqueous to flow through and may be undertaken prophylactically in individuals at risk of angle closure glaucoma.
3. Argon laser PRP (see above) is used in cases of glaucoma secondary to neovascular disease – usually after a central retinal vein occlusion which may lead to rubeosis (new vessels on the iris).

After Cataract Surgery

1. YAG laser is used to make a hole in the membrane behind the lens implant in cases where this membrane thickens and reduces acuity – YAG capsulotomy (Fig. 4.15c).

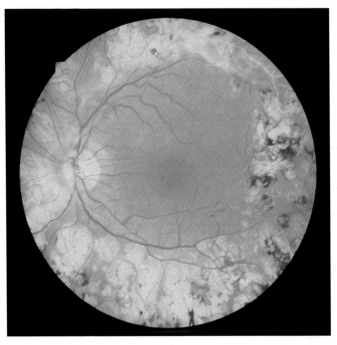

Fig. 10.3 Pan retinal photoablation – the burns may become pigmented with time – note how the central retina is avoided.

2. Laser is not used to remove a cataract – although this technology is under development – an ultrasound probe is usually used (phaco-emulsification, see p. 170).

Chapter 11

Eye Drops and Drugs

Patients frequently present with eye problems that are already being treated, but fail to bring their medications and have no knowledge of the treatment they are on.

This chapter incorporates:

1. List of commonly used eye drops.
2. Common regimes for various conditions (these are also detailed in the appropriate chapter dealing with these conditions).
3. Brief information on individual drops.

COMMON EYE DROPS AND DRUGS

Antibiotic Drops (Figs 11.1–11.3)

Chloramphenicol, Chloromycetin, Sno Phenicol	chloramphenicol 0.5%
Exocin	ofloxacin 0.3%
Ciloxan	ciprofloxacin 0.3%
Fucithalmic	fusidic acid 1% gel
Genticin, Garamycin	gentamicin hydrochloride 0.3%

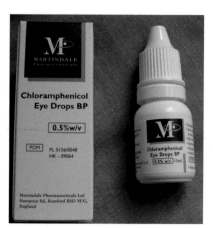

Fig. 11.1 Chloramphenicol eye drops. Courtesy of Martindale Pharmaceuticals.

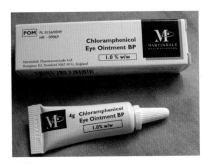

Fig. 11.2a Chloramphenicol eye ointment. Courtesy of Martindale Pharmaceuticals.

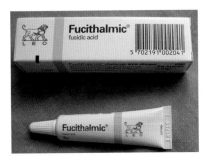

Fig. 11.2b Fucithalmic – fusidic acid. Courtesy of Leo Pharmaceuticals.

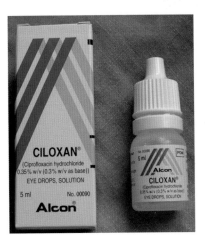

Fig. 11.3 Ciloxan. Courtesy of Alcon Pharmaceuticals.

Antibiotic Ointments

Chloramphenicol, Chloromycetin	chloramphenicol 1%
Aureomycin	chlortetracycline hydrochloride 1%

Antivirals (Fig. 11.4)

Zovirax	aciclovir 3%

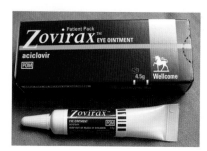

Fig. 11.4 Zovirax – aciclovir. Courtesy of GlaxoSmithKline.

Steroid Drops (Figs 11.5, 11.6)

Pred Forte	prednisolone acetate 1%
Maxidex	dexamethasone 0.1%
Betnesol	betamethasone sodium phosphate 0.1%
Predsol	prednisolone sodium phosphate 0.5%
FML	fluoromethalone 0.1%
	polyvinyl alcohol 1.4%
Vexol	rimexolone 1%

Hayfever and Allergy Related

Rapitil	nedocromil sodium 2%
Alomide	lodoxamide 0.1%
Opticrom	sodium cromoglicate 2%
Otrivine-Antistin	antazoline sulfate 0.5% + xylometazoline hydrochloride 0.05%
Opatanol	olopatadine

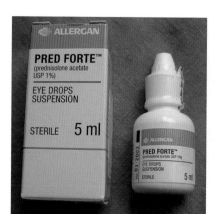

Fig. 11.5 Prednisolone eye drop suspension. Courtesy of Allergan Inc.

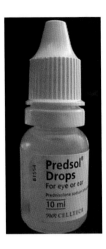

Fig. 11.6   Predsol drops – prednisolone sodium phosphate. Courtesy of Celltech Group Plc.

Glaucoma (Figs 11.7–11.9)

Xalatan	latanoprost 0.005%
Betoptic	betaxolol 0.5%
Timoptol, Timolol	timolol 0.25%, 0.5%
Betagan	levobunolol hydrochloride 0.5%
	polyvinyl alcohol 1.4%
Cosopt	dorzolamide 2%, timolol 0.5%
Alphagan	brimonidine tartrate 0.2%
Pilocarpine	pilocarpine hydrochloride
Diamox tablet, Diamox SR capsule	acetazolamide 250 mg

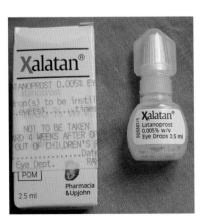

Fig. 11.7   Xalatan – latanoprost eye drops. Courtesy of Pharmacia Corporation.

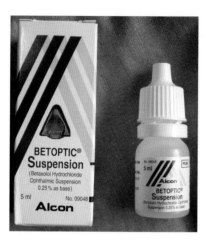

Fig. 11.8 Betoptic suspension. Courtesy of Alcon Pharmaceuticals.

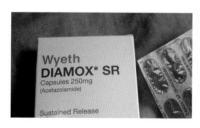

Fig. 11.9 Diamox – acetazolamide. Copyright Wyeth and used with permission.

Pupil Dilators (Fig. 11.10)

Mydriacyl	tropicamide 0.5%, 1%
Mydrilate	cyclopentolate hydrochloride 0.5%
Phenylephrine	phenylephrine hydrochloride 2.5% 10%
Atropine	atropine sulfate 1%
Homatropine	homatropine hydrobromide 1%

Lubricant Drops (Fig. 11.11)

GelTears, Viscotears	polyacrylic acid 0.2%
Hypromellose	hypromellose 0.3%
Tears Naturale	dextran 70 0.1%, hypromellose 0.3%
Artificial Tears minims	hydroxyethylcellulose 0.44%
Liquifilm Tears	polyvinyl alcohol 1.4%

Lubricant Ointment

Lacri-Lube	white soft and liquid paraffin
Ilube	acetylcysteine 5%, hypromellose 0.35%

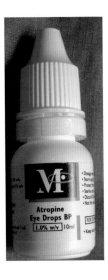

Fig. 11.10   Atropine eye drops. Courtesy of Martindale Pharmaceuticals.

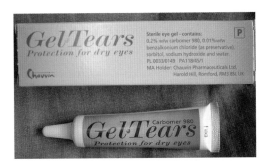

Fig. 11.11   GelTears. Courtesy of Bausch & Lomb UK Ltd.

Anesthetic Drops (Fig. 11.12)

Proxymetacaine	proxymetacaine hydrochloride 0.5%
Proxymetacaine and Fluorescein	as above with fluorescein 0.25%
Lignocaine and Fluorescein	lidocaine hydrochloride 4% and fluorescein sodium 0.25%
Benoxinate	oxybuprocaine hydrochloride 0.4%
Amethocaine	tetracaine hydrochloride 0.5%

Eye Stains (Figs 11.12, 11.13)

Fluorescein	fluorescein sodium 1–2%

Appropriate treatment including dosage and duration is detailed in each section of the book as required.

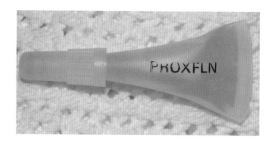

Fig. 11.12 Proxymetacaine and fluorescein combined. Courtesy of Bausch & Lomb UK Ltd.

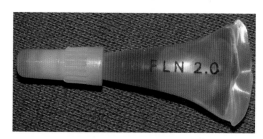

Fig. 11.13 Fluorescein 2%. Courtesy of Bausch & Lomb UK Ltd.

COMMON POSTOPERATIVE REGIMES

Regimes vary. The following are common.

Cataract Surgery

Steroid drops 4 weeks
1. Pred Forte or Maxidex or Betnesol – 4 times daily, 4 weeks then stop.

Antibiotic drops 1–4 weeks
2. Chloramphenicol – 4 times daily, 4 weeks then stop.
or
3. Exocin – 4 times daily, 1 week then stop.

Glaucoma Surgery (Trabeculectomy)

As for cataract surgery above with the addition of:
Dilating drop (not always used)

1. Mydrilate – 3 times daily, 2 weeks then stop.
or
2. Atropine – 2 times daily, 2 weeks, then stop.

Squint Surgery

Various postoperative regimes
Antibiotic alone
Combination antibiotic and steroid
No treatment

1. Chloramphenicol drops or ointment – 3 times daily, 2 weeks then stop.
or
2. Betnesol–N – 3 times daily, 2 weeks then stop.
Note: this option is not commonly used.
or
3. No treatment – common in non-complex cases.

Retinal Detachment Surgery

As for glaucoma surgery above
Atropine is usually used as the dilating agent
Oral analgesia as required.

Laser Refractive Surgery

1. Predsol – 3 times daily for one week.
2. Chloramphenicol – 3 times daily for one week.
3. Combination Predsol-N (neomycin) may be used.
4. Artificial tears 4 times daily – for up to 3 months.

Dacryocystorhinostomy – DCR (For Watering Eyes)

1. No treatment post op.
or
2. Chloramphenicol drops – 4 times daily, 2 weeks then stop.
occasionally with
3. Betnesol drops – 4 times daily, 2 weeks then stop.
Note: these may also be used nasally in endonasal DCRs. Use separate bottles.
4. Oral antibiotic, e.g. Magnapen 500 mg, 4 times daily, 5 days then stop.

Note: usually used only in infective cases, e.g. abscess drainage.

BRIEF NOTES ON EACH COMMON DRUG

Antibiotics

Chloramphenicol
Broad spectrum, bacteriostatic only. Occasional allergic response. Frequency four times daily but can increase to hourly. First-line treatment in simple conjunctivitis. Only very rarely associated with aplastic anemia.

Exocin
Broad spectrum, 10 day course only, effective against *Pseudomonas* infections. Frequency four times daily.

Ciloxan
Usually used for corneal ulcers, hourly instillation required initially.

Genticin
Bacteriocidal. More frequent allergic response. Second line if chloramphenicol fails or *Pseudomonas* suspected. Frequency variable from four times daily to hourly.

Fucithalmic
Broad spectrum. Only requires bd application. First-line treatment in simple conjunctivitis. Useful in staphylococcal infections and treatment of blepharitis. Frequency twice daily.

Aureomycin
Use in suspected chlamydial disease – four times daily for 3 weeks. Treat partner.

Antivirals

Zovirax
Use five times daily for minimum of 5 days. Low corneal toxicity compared with other antivirals. Beware not to use skin preparation Zovirax in the eye.

Steroids

All Topical Steroids
1. May cause secondary glaucoma.
2. May complicate and worsen dendritic ulcers.
3. Should only be prescribed if patient is under the care of an ophthalmologist.

Pred Forte
Milky suspension. Potent steroid with high penetration into anterior chamber. Usually four times daily but may be used hourly in severe inflammation. May cause raised intraocular pressure.

Maxidex
Clear solution, otherwise as for Pred Forte above.

Betnesol
Less potent than Maxidex. Usually four times daily.

Predsol
Less potent than the above. Very weak concentrations may be used long term in corneal scarring due to old viral keratitis. Frequency variable from four times daily to one drop every alternate day.

FML
Less potent and less commonly used. Lower risk of raising intraocular pressure than other steroids.

Hayfever Related

Rapitil, Opatanol
Fast onset of action in comparison to Opticrom. Frequency two to four times daily.

Opticrom
Can take 3 weeks before taking effect. Usual frequency four times daily. Long-term use, but may be restricted to hayfever season.

Alomide
Fast onset of action. Usual frequency four times daily.

Glaucoma

1. **Patients should not stop anti-glaucoma treatment unless instructed to do so by an ophthalmologist or physician.**
2. **Breathlessness may occur with beta blockers – see below.**

Timoptol, Betoptic, Betagan – These are Beta Blockers
Contraindicated in chronic obstructive airways disease and heart block. Frequency twice daily.

Xalatan
Highly effective. Rarely associated with uveitis. May cause change in iris color (increased pigmentation). Frequency once daily.

Pilocarpine
Causes pupil miosis (small pupil). Headaches and poor vision in the dark common initially. Infrequent allergic reaction (local effect). Frequency usually four times daily.

Propine
Causes pupil dilatation (enlarged pupil). Allergic conjunctivitis not uncommon. Frequency twice daily. Less frequently used now.

Alphagan
Used if beta blockers contraindicated. Local allergic response not uncommon. Frequency twice daily.

Ganda

Now withdrawn. Rarely associated with uveitis.

Diamox

IV – 500 mg powder dissolved in 10 ml water for injections. For rapid intraocular pressure reduction.

PO – 250–500 mg tablets. Usual maximum 1 g per day. Slow release preparation available, frequency twice daily.

Pupil Dilators (and Ciliary Muscle Relaxants)

Mydrilate

Duration up to 12 hours. Will cause blurring particularly for reading. Advise against driving after instillation. Beware in the elderly – particularly if longsighted (check glasses – lenses correcting long sight act as magnifying lenses) as you may precipitate angle closure glaucoma – this is however rare. Usual frequency twice daily.

Atropine

Duration up to 2 weeks. Allergy may occur. Usually used in severe uveitis. Occasionally used in children to measure for spectacles however beware of systemic effects – tachycardia, flushing, dry mouth and delerium. Lethal doses in young children may be reached using eye drops.

Homatropine

Infrequently used. As for Mydrilate – but has longer duration of action.

Lubricants

Hypromellose, Tears Naturelle, Artificial Tears, Liquifilm

All may be used for symptomatic relief as frequently as necessary – even half hourly. Allergy to preservative may occur.

Lacri-Lube

Ointment used in addition to drops in severe dry eye or recurrent corneal erosion. Often just used before bed as blurs vision transiently and may be unsightly giving an oily appearance around eyes.

Ilube

Infrequently used. Discomfort if used long term. Used to dissolve excess mucus in tear film – usually with dry eyes. Frequency twice to four times daily.

Anesthetics

Do not issue topical anesthetics to patients – frequent instillation may cause epithelial damage, mask corneal damage and slows corneal epithelial healing.

Proxymetacaine
Virtually painless instillation – particularly good with children. Causes little corneal epithelial change – hence useful during cataract surgery.

Benoxinate
More comfortable than amethocaine, less comfortable than proxymetacaine. Warn patient it will sting for 30 seconds or so.

Amethocaine
Uncomfortable for 30 seconds – warn patient. Repeated use may lead to extensive corneal and conjunctival epithelial defects which are extremely painful and slow to heal.

Stains

Fluorescein
Drop form or dried onto a strip (Fluoret). Use sparingly. If concentrated, i.e. 2% in minims dropper, it will not fluoresce under cobalt blue light, thus corneal defects may be missed. Dilute with a drop of saline if required.

Index

References to figures and other non-textual materials are in italics. American spellings are used.